Mean Girls, Meaner Women

Understanding Why Women Backstab, Betray, and Trash-Talk Each Other and How to Heal

Dr. Erika Holiday and Dr. Joan I. Rosenberg

Authors' Note
Any references or resemblance to any persons or organizations, whether living or dead, existing or defunct, is purely coincidental.

Disclaimer and/or Legal Notices:
While all attempts have been made to verify information provided in this book and its ancillary materials, neither the authors nor publisher assumes any responsibility for errors, inaccuracies, or omissions.

The authors of this book are not physicians, and the ideas, procedures, and suggestions in this book are not psychological advice or counsel nor is it intended to take the place of medical or psychological advice from trained psychological professionals. Readers are advised to consult qualified health professionals regarding treatment of medical or psychological problems and before adopting the suggestions in this book. The authors and publisher disclaim any liability arising directly or indirectly from use of this book. Neither the publisher nor the authors take any responsibility for any possible consequences from any treatment, action, or application of exercises to any person reading or following the information in this book.

Visit www.amazon.com to order additional copies.

For my mother,
Eva

My father,
Karim

My brother,
Donny

For my mother,
Lorraine

My sister,
Susan

My brother,
Jay

And in loving memory of my father,
Theodore

Contents

Chapter I

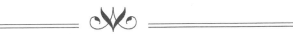

Introduction

Erika's Story

During the summer of 2004 I boarded a plane at Los Angeles International Airport headed to Europe for a family vacation. My brother, mother, and I traveled together for our last visit with my grandmother—she died the following year. My mother and I sat next to each other and my brother was seated nearby, though he remained in plain view. As soon as we were seated, the female flight attendant wasted no time greeting my brother and tending to him. Yet there was no greeting or response for me or my mother. Minutes later she brought my brother a Diet Coke and asked him if he was okay—still no attention to us. As I watched the flight attendant repeatedly cater to my brother, I wondered if she was purposely ignoring me and my mom or if we were perhaps assigned to a different flight attendant.

This same story unfolded for quite some time. We watched my brother being catered to . . . Soda? Pillow? Blanket? Any efforts on our part to get the flight attendant's attention were met with her disdain. A common story perhaps, but our experience nonetheless.

My mother and I were bewildered and we seemed invisible to the flight attendant. We discussed her rude and dismissive behavior and wondered what we did that elicited such a negative response from her. Being routinely ignored by the flight attendant led us into conversation about the ways women often mistreat other women. We traded stories about our own friendships, and my mother told me stories that I had never heard before, many having to do with her youth and how she felt that many of her friends were hateful toward and competitive with her over beauty, boyfriends, and popularity.

Then we browsed through tabloid magazines I had brought on the plane. We took note of how many magazines were filled with accounts of competition between women, not healthy competition, but nasty and hostile stories with headlines of "Catfight"...

"Betrayal". . . and "Backstabbed." We had a lengthy and spirited exchange as we talked about our life experiences, especially involving ways in which females hurt each other. Despite so many advances over the past thirty years based on the Women's Movement, even a generation later, I too experienced similar competitive and hurtful behavior from other girls and women. Had nothing changed?

During that same summer I was expected to begin writing my doctoral thesis[1] for graduate school. I had run through several possible topics with Joan, who was serving as my mentor for the project, yet she had rejected all my previous ideas. She wanted me to choose a topic about which I felt passionate, yet was unique to the field of psychology. My flight to Europe provided the answer. I couldn't stop thinking about how often I felt betrayed and hurt by other females. I began reliving many vivid memories of being in school where I was teased or excluded by other girls because I didn't wear the right kind of clothes, hang out with the right kinds of friends, or sometimes for really nothing at all.

I felt compelled to write my thesis on women oppressing women so I could explain how women become women who hurt, betray, backstab, or "trash-talk" other women. There is extensive research on oppression by men toward women, but I had never read any literature about female-to-female oppression. This issue had certainly not been discussed in any of my psychology texts!

And then I started searching . . . overall, little was to be found on this issue. I felt frustrated and totally confused. How could I write a thesis on a topic that had such limited research? Despite the dearth of information, I struggled to understand how a girl develops into the kind of woman who hurts another woman. Imagine my further confusion as I explained my frustration finding research and Joan's response was to be excited. I clearly remember how animated she became as she explained how important it was to explore a topic that could educate women about an issue to which most women can relate yet few openly and seriously discuss.

On the basis of her own experiences, as a child and as an adult, addressing this topic was of great import to her too. I asked her to join me as co-author; her suggestions and guidance contributed significantly to my work.

About the Book

At least weekly there are media reports of nasty feuds and hurtful conflicts between women. Consider the ones highlighted most over the past couple of years—Lauren Conrad and Heidi Montag, Paris Hilton and Nicole Ritchie, or the very public feud between Rosie O'Donnell and Elizabeth Hasselback. It's hard to know who to believe. Despite the reports, few media venues seriously address meanness between women.

When women are asked if they were ever emotionally hurt or bullied by other girls, or by women, they immediately recount episodes with remarkable clarity, as if it happened yesterday. These experiences remain unforgettable, and for many women the hurt leaves permanent emotional scars. Does this sound familiar? It did to the women who attended our presentations and trainings and to our psychotherapy clients.

Every time we broached the issue of hurtful behavior between women, women were eager to disclose their own stories; whether from childhood or adulthood, they detailed how girls and women had hurt them. They felt confused and concerned about the issue themselves and said they found few women who would talk openly about this problem; there were no obvious resources or people to whom they could turn for help.

Women hurt, betray, backstab, and "trash-talk" each other. We know from personal experiences and from the many stories told to us by other girls and women. They express a sincere interest in understanding why women hurt each other. The answer is not a simple one; this phenomenon occurs based on a confluence of countless different factors.

The purpose for writing this book includes raising awareness about this issue and helping girls and women who have experienced oppression or who oppress others change the nature of their relationships. The intent is to help women develop relationships that are stronger, more collaborative, more authentically open, and less bound by the constrictions of cultural norms about gender. Women can bond together for the pure joy this connection brings and for the social good to which it can lead. Suggestions for helping enhance women's relationships and a variety of other resources are provided at the end of the book.

We want women to connect with each other in nurturing and loving ways—to promote positive changes for all girls and women. We encourage women to have open conversations with each other about their relationships, especially when hurtful, angry, or competitive feelings are involved. Perhaps this book can act as a catalyst for broaching challenging issues and for facilitating increasingly honest discussions between women. It can similarly serve as a guide for parents or teachers. Mothers can help their daughters to think more critically about the societal messages bombarding young girls regarding how they should behave; choose gender behaviors more congruent with their true selves; decrease self-hating and emotionally disconnecting behaviors; learn to manage angry and competitive feelings more effectively; and establish closer bonds with girls as they grow up.

The concepts and ideas for this book originated in the work completed for my (Erika's) doctoral thesis. Highlighted are aspects of life to which women are exposed that include societal and cultural factors, psychological processes, and brain, evolutionary, and media influences that affect first a girl's and then a woman's choices and behavior.

We look at the gender roles girls most often adopt and how women are socialized into these particular roles. Likewise we describe a variety of social factors that impact how girls are raised and the societal implications these influences can have on women. How our media-saturated culture has significantly influenced girls and women is considered along with information that explains oppression, the effects of oppression, and social pressures experienced in groups.

Our view of women oppressing women emerges out of and is adapted from research on relational aggression previously conducted on children and adolescents, conceptual writing about racism and oppression, and from our numerous conversations during groups, presentations, and workshops. Though this book is not the result of a formal research endeavor, information was drawn from a combination of informal conversations, interviews, workshop/presentations, client sessions and groups, with over 450 girls and 350 women from varied ages, cultural backgrounds, and ethnicities. I (Erika) conducted several presentations with public high school girls in the Los Angeles area; attendance ranged from 70 to 120 girls at each presentation. More than fifteen workshops that ranged from two to four hours in length were conducted with women; attendees at several of the workshops were psychologists, social workers, marriage and family therapists, and graduate psychology students. The size of the workshops ranged from ten to forty participants. Workshop topics and activities included exercises exploring a woman's experience with oppressive female behavior; defining women oppressing women; brain, evolutionary, gender socializing, and media influences; and suggestions for changing hurtful behavior between women. Remaining information was drawn from our clinical experience and conversations with over thirty female clients.

We look at both sides of the issue and describe a woman's experience as either a victim or perpetrator of hurtful female behavior. Women were asked to talk about why they gossip about, hurt, turn their backs on, or betray each other in an effort to understand what makes so many women question the honesty and authenticity of their relationships with each other. Many of their stories are incorporated throughout the book.

The Key Link: Self-Hatred

The path a girl travels from childhood to adulthood that leads her to hurt women is one carved out by self-hate; rigid gender roles for girls and women; damaging societal and media messages about female behavior; psychological, biological, and evolutionary pressures; intense competition, and hidden effects of female to female oppression. The complex interplay between these psychological and social pressures are as simultaneously intriguing and compelling as they are unfair, unjust, and destructive.

Hurtful behaviors that occur between adult women parallel similar behavior seen in girls. These hurtful behaviors emerge out of an experience of self-hatred and *self-hatred is the key link* between girls' early hurtful behavior toward each other and women who oppress women. A woman with a strong sense of self and high self-esteem is much less likely to hurt others.

Consider the ways girls and women are portrayed by the media in United States culture. Generally, they are socialized into several impossible double binds and they are discouraged from directly expressing anger. A double bind occurs when contradictory demands are made on an individual, so that no matter which demand is followed, the individual's response will be construed as incorrect. The influence of these double binds combine with pressures to conform and behave in a stereotyped female manner; together these forces serve as a strong means of disempowering women so that ultimately women do not rebel against something they believe cannot be changed. Believing and engaging in stereotyped female behavior often leaves women participating in their own oppression.

John Jost, a social psychologist, suggests that members of oppressed groups often internalize aspects of their oppression and come to believe in their imposed inferiority.[2] Though women frequently have a hard time admitting they experience themselves as being inferior to men, largely this appears to be true. Phyllis Chesler, a psychologist known for her writing about women's issues, described how many women have internalized societal messages that undermine their own self-worth and how societal devaluation of women creates the tendency for women to devalue "other" women.[3] Think about this: **each time a woman devalues another woman, she inevitably devalues herself.**

Speaking of women undermining their own self worth . . . does a woman really enjoy wearing four-inch heels, sexy thongs, and tight Spanx, or did she internalize societal messages suggesting to her that she is supposed to love wearing these things? These and countless other similar messages are so ingrained in our culture that women believe that these interests or behaviors are natural and inevitable. The point is not so much about four-inch heels, it is more about how a woman makes decisions about what she believes and how she feels and acts. How a woman responds to cultural and peer pressures has implications for how she relates to other women.

Unfortunately, when women do not think critically about cultural beliefs and messages or peer pressure, they participate unwittingly in their own oppression. Given the social pressures that women experience and the likelihood that many women haven't seriously reflected upon these pressures, one possibility is that women are frustrated and angry about often unacknowledged oppression. Many women then unknowingly turn their anger and aggression onto other women.

Breaking the Code of Silence Between Women

Women often keep a "code of silence" about conflict and about competitive and angry feelings between them. These feelings are often turned inward, remaining unexpressed, or they are expressed through indirect hurtful attacks on the other woman. It is common for a woman to first recognize how she has been hurt by a woman. Later she may acknowledge having been cruel to other women.

Most women eventually identify with both sides of cruelty—that of being a victim and of being a perpetrator—but because verbal aggression is not generally perceived the same as physical aggression, women often "get away with" hurting other women. These subtle and blatant attacks keep women at an emotional distance from each other. The result is that authenticity and genuineness within women's relationships are lost. Exposing how hurtful women can be to each other creates an opportunity to address issues between them that remain insidious, festering in the darkness of silence, that have served as hidden forces keeping women emotionally distant from and untrusting of each other.

Your Relationships with Girls and Women

Awareness can help you make clearer and more informed choices. Be reflective about your own life whether you were the target of others' cruelty, whether you stood by and watched, feeling confused about what to do, or if you were a girl or woman who treated (or treats) others in a mean or hurtful manner. Jot down some thoughts as they come to you.

Start by going back and thinking about your childhood and adolescence, specifically about your relationships with your peers.

- Did you go through childhood and adolescence without being hurt by girls?
- Were you picked on / ridiculed / taunted / excluded / shamed by your peers during childhood and adolescence?
- As you grew up did you feel like you never fit in with other girls?
- What was the impact on you if you were the object of others' hurtful word or actions?
- Were you a girl who hurt other girls? How did you go about hurting them?
- Did you pick on girls by excluding, gossiping about, or physically hurting them?
- What do you think prompted you to behave hurtfully toward others if you did so (or, in general, why do you think this even happens)?
- What are your thoughts about your experience as a child and adolescent?

Now think about your adulthood and what you experience and the ways you behave now . . .

- Do you continue to be the object of women's hurtful words/actions?
- How is it that others see you as a target of their hateful or excluding behavior?
- Do you engage in gossiping about other women, saying mean things to women, or participate in hurtful, cruel, or excluding behaviors toward women?
- What are your thoughts about the degree of emotional closeness or emotional distance you feel towards women in your life?
- Who is close to you? Who do you feel distant from?
- Do the women in your life know the "real" you?

Chapter II

Smackdown!

Types of Aggressive Behavior

Many of you may remember the movie *Mean Girls* [1] based on the non-fiction book *Queen Bees and Wannabes* by Rosalind Wiseman. [2] Wiseman's book describes how female high school social cliques operate and the effect they can have on girls. Briefly, the movie is about a sixteen-year-old girl (Cady Heron / *Lindsay Lohan*) who lives in an affluent area of suburban Chicago after having moved from Africa where she was raised and home schooled by her parents. She attends a public high school and is confronted by rules and restrictions at school as she struggles to fit in with her new peers. She meets Janis Ian (*Lizzy Caplan*) and Damian (*Daniel Franzese*), two students who help her learn about the school cliques and social hierarchy. The movie centers on how she is bullied by three spiteful girls (Karen Smith / *Amanda Seyfield*, Gretchen Wieners / *Lacey Chabert*, and Regina George / *Rachel McAdams*) in the most popular clique, "The Plastics," adopts their behavior, and, by the movie's end, learns how to have caring and healthier relationships with her friends.

Hurtful behaviors between the girls seen in the *Mean Girls* movie illustrate different types of aggression. There was *direct* (Regina punching a girl in the face), *indirect* (Regina spreading rumors about Janis' sexuality during their middle school years), *relational* (Cady is able to manipulate Gretchen and Karen into getting angry at Regina, so that eventually Regina is kicked out of The Plastics clique), and *social* aggression (Cady is introduced to "The Burn Book," in which insulting comments are made about the other girls and some teachers in the school). The different kinds of hurtful behavior are explained below.

DIRECT AGGRESSION:

harm delivered in a face-to-face situation

Main aim: inflicting harm

(Archer & Coyne, 2005)

Another example of *direct aggression* comes from the *The House Bunny* (2008) movie that includes scenes where women can be seen punching each other in the arm or the breast.[3]

INDIRECT AGGRESSION:

"harm delivered circuitously" or "behind the back"

Main aim: intent is to adversely affect one's social
standing

(Björkqvist, Österman, & Kaukiainen, 1992, p. 52;
Björkqvist, et al., 2001, p. 113)

The main consequences of *indirect aggression* are to *exclude, negatively impact, or manipulate the reputation of someone by lowering her social standing* within her clique.[4] An example of such aggression can be seen in *The House Bunny* movie. Sienna (*Leslie Del Rosario*) and Shelley (*Anna Faris*) are two women living in the Playboy Mansion with Hugh Hefner and vying for a spot as an upcoming centerfold in Playboy magazine. Shelley receives a letter from Hugh Hefner telling her she must move out of the mansion immediately. Shelley follows directions and moves out, only to find out much later that Sienna had written the letter so she could assure her own spot in the magazine. Sienna's letter, written behind Shelley's back, was intended to knock her out of the "bunny" clique. It effectively drums her out of the house and out of any opportunity to be the centerfold.

Bridget, a young woman attending one of our workshops, described how she wanted to be student body president several years ago during her senior year of high school. She recounted how she confided these dreams to her best friend, Lily. Little did Bridget know that Lily had actually been quite envious of Bridget's motivation, popularity, and accomplishments. Without Bridget's awareness, Lily began positioning herself to be voted as student body president herself and was spreading vicious rumors about Bridget so that she would not be elected. This caused a huge conflict and rift in their friendship, and their mutual friends started taking sides. A third girl, Gillian, ended up being selected instead leaving neither Bridget nor Lily in that role. Though Bridget was left extremely disappointed and confused by what happened with Gillian being selected, Lily didn't really care. Lily's intent was simply to "take Bridget down," without Bridget being able to figure out how it happened and who did it to her.

By using indirect means of aggression, an aggressor can remain unknown to the victim, and, by remaining unidentifiable, she is able to avoid possible counterattack. Using the example, Bridget had no way to defend herself because the perpetrator, Lily, remained invisible. What is particularly advantageous to the aggressor is that she is able to either hide her identity, often through a third person (getting someone else to say mean things to the targeted victim), or to deny hostile/aggressive intent so she can pretend the attack was not aggressive at all.

> ## SOCIAL AGGRESSION:
>
> "the manipulation of group acceptance through alienation, ostracism, or character defamation"
>
> (Cairns, Cairns, Neckerman, Ferguson, & Gariepy, 1989, p. 323)

Emma, one of Erika's past clients, related a hurtful incident from her high school days. She was a high school cheerleader and had been dating Mark for three years. Heather was a fellow cheerleader who began showing Mark that she was interested in him by calling him and passing notes to him in class. Emma was so angry at Heather's flirtatious behavior that she started a rumor about Heather being a whore and a slut. Within a few days, Heather got wind of what was being said about her and presumed Emma was the source of the rumor, yet there was no way of proving it. There was little Heather could do for "damage control," yet she made efforts to talk with her peers to minimize the cost to her reputation. While Emma said she deeply regretted her actions at that time, there were no consequences for her. Heather's reputation, however, was damaged by Emma's hostile action.

Dr. Marion Underwood, a clinical psychologist who specializes in work with children, suggested that social aggression could be used to describe obvious and hidden forms of relational manipulation and also harmful nonverbal behaviors (e.g. rolling the eyes or giving dirty or disapproving looks).[5] *Social aggression* has also been used to broadly describe indirect and relational aggression and all types of manipulative and deceitful behavior.[6]

> ### RELATIONAL AGGRESSION:
>
> "overt or covert behaviors that harm others through damage (or the threat of damage) to particular relationships or to feelings of acceptance, friendship, or group inclusion."
>
> Main aim: the intent to harm either a given relationship or group membership
>
> (Crick & Grotpeter, 1995; Crick et al., 1999, p. 77)

Annie, a woman in her late thirties and one of Joan's clients, described herself as a conscientious, hard-working, and well-respected lawyer in her corporation. Others would describe her at the "top of her game," something her supervisor, Kelly, despised, because Kelly was, as she herself had described, the self-proclaimed "queen bee." Annie easily related how she had been kept from plum assignments and committees, and in fact had been told by Kelly that had Kelly had the choice in hiring, Annie would never have been hired onto her team. Kelly also actively teamed up with another professional within their corporation to get Annie demoted from a recent promotion, taking her efforts even a step further by "bad-mouthing" Annie to the CEO of the organization and ensuring that Annie would not be able to comfortably retain her position. All of these efforts left Kelly with the upper hand, thus retaining her self-proclaimed "queen-bee" status and position.

Relational aggression often involves *highly manipulative acts expressed through hostile, aggressive, coercive, or controlling behavior* (for instance, threatening to break off the friendship if the person won't comply with the request—a situation that often sounds like "if you really liked me, you would do what I wanted"). Kelly's refusal to give Annie good assignments or committee positions was quite controlling, and her comment about never wanting to hire her was clearly hostile to Annie.

When it comes to understanding relational aggression, it does not matter whether the hurtful actions were obvious or hidden, nor does it matter whether the victim knows the person causing the hurt. Throughout this book, we use the phrase *relational aggression* or *relationally aggressive behavior* to discuss hurtful behaviors between girls or women.

Indirect aggression is intended to *affect someone's social standing* or it is intended to hurt the person's reputation; *relational aggression*, by contrast, feeds off the importance of relationships, as the focus is to *manipulate the friendship or the dyad* itself. [7, 8] The bottom line is that whether a woman experiences or engages in direct, indirect, relational, or social aggression, they all have the same underlying theme—one female is hurting another female.

Cyberbullying:
Taking Hurt to a Whole New Level

Sophie, a twenty-year-old college student attending one of our talks, described how she had been humiliated by girls while in high school. A photo of Sophie in her underwear had been posted on the Internet. The pictures were posted on MySpace, one of the social networking sites on the Internet, where others could make harassing comments about her or even rate her, which added to her humiliation. The worst part for Sophie was that she initially thought that her friends might have taken the photo of her. Later she learned that girls from a different clique took a picture of her while she was changing in the girl's locker room. Sophie described how she became depressed because of this incident and felt isolated and withdrawn from her friends, family, and school activities.

Sophie is not alone. The National Crime Prevention Council (NCPC) stated that six out of every ten American teen students witness *bullying* in school at least once a day. Bullying includes all forms of aggressive behavior, whether it occurs repeatedly or just once. It affects nearly one in three American school children in grades six through ten. Eighty-three percent of *girls* and 79 percent of boys report experiencing harassment in schools.[9]

Today's bully may be stylistically more advanced than the bullies of the past. Most girls grow up with access to a number of technological advances, particularly in American culture. Availability of these resources has resulted in attacks on others through new mediums (e.g. computer and wireless phone, text or video messaging) known as *cyberbullying.*

Cyberbullies can use e-mail, instant messaging (IM), text messaging, cell phone cameras, and websites to hurt and humiliate other girls. Information on w*iredsafety.org,* a website dedicated to educating and raising awareness about cyberbullying and promoting computer safety while online, states that 90 percent of students have had their feelings hurt online and 75 percent have visited a website bashing another student.[10]

Researchers have found that girls rule when it comes to online bullying. Nearly one-third of eighth-grade girls, as reported in one survey, described being bullied online in the last two months, compared with 10 percent of boys.[11] During a workshop I (Erika) recently conducted on relational aggression with seventy-five high school girls, I asked how many girls had visited websites, chat rooms, or text messaged other girls as a means of intentionally hurting other girls. The prevalence of online bullying is high— nearly half of the girls raised their hands.

Not only do girls and women visit websites or chat rooms, they create websites with the sole intention of harm. One such website was built by a woman to degrade and demean the popular TV host Rachel Ray, a woman with a quick rise to fame. On the website, Rachel is called a variety of names, her family history is mocked, and her creations devalued. It appears others are quite jealous of her success. How else might we explain some woman building a website to demean another woman?

Rachel Simmons, in her book *Odd Girl Out*, discusses how girls use anonymous means of attack so that they can never be found out.[12] This is true for cyberbullying as well. On the computer, unfortunately, one can easily steal someone else's name or pose as a different person while insulting and defaming an identified target.

Jenni, a fourteen year old participant at one of the in-school workshops, told us that she and her friends in her eighth-grade class were already using the Internet to gain popularity among their friends. She described how she and her friends would flirt with boys online to get them involved in their schemes, which included ganging up on other girls in school by spreading false rumors about those girls on their My Space pages.

Since young girls like Jenni have grown up with the Internet, their technological skills have provided them an outlet that many women did not experience growing up. Girls like Jenni can easily hurt and betray other girls without having to be face-to-face with who is being hurt.

The television show *Primetime* aired a special on September 12, 2006 called "Mean Girls and Cyberbullying."[13] ABC News worked with the Brigham Young University child development researchers and iSafe's Schroeder to develop an experiment using technology as weapons that looked closely into teenage competition. They found the girls were skilled and technologically advanced at using cyberspace as a means of hurting others. The girls used their sexuality and means of attacking others to gain power and reach the top of their social hierarchy.

These researchers found that the "safety" of anonymity allowed the girls to feel like they could act in ways that they normally wouldn't if they were face-to-face with another girl. Once the experiment was completed, many of the girls related that they couldn't believe how mean they acted, and they described feeling remorseful for behaving so cruelly to others.

One way for girls to take revenge on other girls is to videotape their fights and then post them on the Internet. Typing "girlfight" on YouTube.com yields thousands of search results. Girls are using the Internet to cause hurt and long-lasting emotional pain, as girls attack each other through their relationships. Examples also abound from popular culture.

Consider how many girls and women who hold pageant titles have made headlines recently for their "unladylike" behaviors. Elyse Umemoto, the second runner-up for the 2007 Miss America Pageant, was attacked in the press in July 2008 after she was shown on the popular website TMZ engaging in various forms of "un-sweet" behavior. The photo shows her in her bra and underwear and wearing her crown while playing beer pong, flipping off the camera, and making suggestive hand signs. Elyse stated that a friend had leaked her personal photos and that she felt deeply hurt and betrayed by the action.

Another example involves six Florida girls who were tried as adults in early 2008; they could be sentenced to life in prison for their alleged roles in the videotaped beating of another teen girl.[14] The suspects ranged in age from fourteen to eighteen and all face charges of kidnapping, a first-degree felony. The sixteen-year-old victim was shown being punched, kneed, and slapped by other girls. The victim was hospitalized as a result. The girls showed no remorse and laughed as they were arrested and booked. Allegedly the girls were retaliating for insults the victim posted on the Internet.

Cyberbullying brings hostility to a whole new level. Not only do girls physically attack other girls, they post content on the Internet to humiliate the victim further. The attacks "show" how "powerful" the girls are, without concern for how attacks may permanently scar the victim.

Use of the Internet helps persuade and shape people's lives, sometimes with deadly results. The death of St. Louis, Missouri, teenager Megan Meier is a devastating example of relational aggression via the Internet. The mother of Megan's peer created a fake profile on a social networking site. Megan committed suicide after being demeaned, insulted, and rejected by this fictitious person. Countless other examples of hostility and demeaning behavior between women can be found on websites where they are exposed in embarrassing or humiliating situations.

Meanness as a Coping Strategy

Katie, a twenty-seven-year-old workshop participant, told us that when she was in college, she was jealous of her roommate, Amanda, because Amanda was everything Katie felt she was not ... thin, attractive, and smart. Amanda was taking courses required to become a medical doctor, something Katie always had yearned to be, though Katie was unable to master the needed coursework. Katie felt threatened by Amanda's continuing successes, and she described how she realized years later just how jealous she was of Amanda and how she wanted to somehow take away what Amanda had, and the best way she could hurt her was through her words. Katie wanted Amanda to feel as bad as she felt. In an effort to make her look badly in the eyes of their mutual friends, she attempted to defame Amanda by ruining her reputation. Based on their experience as roommates, Katie started spreading rumors that Amanda had contracted a sexually transmitted disease from "sleeping around." This couldn't have been farther from the truth. Once Amanda learned of Katie's dishonest and undercutting behavior, they ceased to be roommates, and Katie lost a friend who she felt truly understood her.

What Katie didn't understand is just how badly she felt about herself. Rather than facing her own insecurities or talking about her feelings directly with Amanda, she took out her anger on the woman who was closest to her. Katie's difficulties experiencing and expressing her genuine feelings and then being mean to Amanda is an example of poor emotional regulation.

To be able to *self-regulate* means being able to pause and self-reflect on thoughts and feelings before acting. Lashing out at someone when angry is poor emotional regulation. If a woman can pause for a few moments, think about her anger, and then talk it out respectfully, she exhibits good self-regulation. Essential elements of "well-being" include being well-intentioned toward others and having the ability to handle feelings well—what psychologists call good *emotional* or *self-regulation*.

Thinking before acting isn't easy. Impulsivity, speed, and instant gratification dictate and drive us. And everything is competitive . . . you have to be faster, better, more regardless of the focus of the competition. Girls and women are under intense and unrelenting pressure to be a certain way in the world—the smartest, thinnest, most attractive, and highly successful. Women often hide parts of themselves because of pressure to be seen a certain way by others. Sometimes these pressures lead a woman to lose sight of who she really is, and the pressures often constrain women from being genuine and authentic with others.

Something to Think About

> Have you ever lashed out at someone else or hurt yourself by being self-destructive (e.g. use of diuretics, laxatives, vomiting, cutting) when you had a hard time feeling angry, sad, frustrated, or disappointed? Any one of these behaviors is an example of poor emotional regulation.

Girls are frequently told to be nice, play nice, and not to perform better than boys. They are more often encouraged to act fearful and withdraw from competitive situations or conflicts, or be passive and dependent rather than independent and strong. They are taught to be less active and not to fight or be physically aggressive. Overall, girls receive distinct messages discouraging them from expressing negative feelings, especially anger.

Even though females have made tremendous progress when it comes to leveling the playing field in a variety of academic disciplines and work arenas, enormous pressures still remain on girls and women to be sweet, kind, and nurturing, as opposed to exhibiting competitiveness or toughness. As a result, girls quickly learn to suppress feelings of anger and hostility rather than express them outwardly.

These messages come at an enormous cost. In the ideal, anger would be directed at whom or what is causing the hurt. Instead there is a tendency for girls and women to keep anger inside and then become self-destructive, or to turn on each other and hurt other girls or women. Given the value women place on relationships with men, there is less tendency for women to take their anger out on men. They highly value relationships with boys and men and sometimes change their behavior in front of them, so behavior between girls and between women must also take relationships with men into consideration.

Emily, one of the women in our groups, talked about her experience growing up in a family that favored her brother and diminished her feelings and any accomplishments she achieved. No one ever noticed or acknowledged the anger and hurt she felt as a child and adolescent, and, as a consequence, no one ever asked about what she felt. Emily said that she was rarely given the "emotional space" to express her feelings, and instead she spent years shutting down on her emotions. Poor coping followed, as Emily said she started binge eating and then purging as a way to handle her anger and other painful feelings, a strategy she knows is all too common for many women. She said she still struggles at times to accurately identify when she is angry, and that expressing her anger at others is a skill she continues to work on and develop. So she may start by using food to cope when she is particularly stressed, until she figures out how best to express herself. Emily also said that once she reached adulthood and was achieving many successes of her own, she found it difficult to feel proud of herself for these accomplishments. She said it has really taken some time for her to fully enjoy the compliments she now receives from her friends for her work.

Anne Conway, a psychologist who has studied boys' and girls' aggression, suggested that if young girls are socialized to inhibit and suppress certain emotions, then this ongoing practice of shutting down feelings, particularly difficult or unpleasant feelings, might result in certain emotional and behavioral deficits for girls.[15] Like Emily, when girls suppress feelings, they may develop poor strategies with which to modulate their feelings, words, or actions.

For instance, if girls are specifically socialized to inhibit anger and aggression, then as girls mature into adult women, they will have fewer strategies to competently experience, modulate, and express anger as they age. If other unpleasant feelings are suppressed as well, girls may end up having fewer and less flexible coping strategies for handling other feelings, including pleasant ones, as a result of all the shutting down. Consequently girls may find it difficult to handle feelings like competitiveness or pride, a situation described by Emily. If Emily had learned to express her feelings instead of turning her anger on herself through food, a practice far too common in our culture, then she might have felt more emotional strength and self-confidence as she matured.

Even though young girls are generally successful controlling emotions and behaviors that involve *physical aggression*, girls may exhibit less success controlling emotions and behaviors that involve *relational aggression*. Constraints that girls are asked to impose over being physically aggressive may inhibit them from developing good strategies later for modulating or handling feelings of anger.

These limits may inadvertently contribute to girls developing relationally aggressive behaviors as one means for expressing anger.[16]

For instance, when there are a few outlets and no flexible strategies for effectively handling unpleasant feelings, girls may instead express anger through hurtful behaviors against other girls as a primary outlet for such feelings. Resorting to hurtful behavior becomes a way to modulate negative emotions, especially when other attempts to handle unpleasant feelings (e.g. anger) have failed.[17]

No one is advocating physical aggression. Yet over-controlling urges to be physical may be one factor that contributes to relational aggression. Strenuous physical exercise or physically demanding sports or activities can serve as a great release of anger or physical aggression.

Sharon Lamb, author of *The Secret Lives of Girls,* also notes that girls have few opportunities to openly express their aggression or anger, so they strike out at other girls in covert ways such as excluding them, gossiping, or damaging reputations.[18] She believes that when girls feel anger toward a boy they do not express it because they feel the boys hold too much power. As a result, girls turn against each other as they compete for boys' attention. So girls go after other girls. She describes it as the weak fighting the weak.[19]

Meanness is a coping strategy, albeit an ineffective and very damaging one. Self-hatred is the link between relationally aggressive behaviors seen in girls through childhood, adolescence, and then into adulthood; the self-hatred emerges out of an absence of genuine personal power and self-efficacy. Meanness then becomes the strategy for increasing self-importance, popularity, or to achieve a desired goal.

Being mean to others is just one strategy, albeit a poor one, for handling uncomfortable feelings. Another outlet, also a poor choice, is to turn unpleasant and angry feelings inward. Clearly, girls and women attempt to cope with unpleasant feelings through countless self-destructive behaviors including anorexia, bulimia, drug use, or other self-destructive acts.

Many girls are unable to deal with their uncomfortable feelings to the point of viciously attacking and hurting other girls, a phenomenon evidenced by a growing number of headlines, articles, and news reports of meanness seen between girls and competitiveness and hostility between women. Societal pressures and the consequences of such pressures suggest that as a society we are not being adequately responsible nor effective at teaching girls how to competently deal with their feelings, especially feelings that involve anger, aggression, competition, or toughness.

Researchers have found that there are long-lasting effects for both the victim and the perpetrators of relationally aggressive behaviors, noting that victims of relational aggression tend to be more depressed, experience anxiety, and have lower self-esteem. [20, 21, 22] Rachel Simmons, author of the book *Odd Girl Out*, describes her interviews with girls and women, some of whom described bullying so severe that they developed ulcers and eating disorders, transferred to other schools, used drugs, or became depressed or suicidal and underwent psychological counseling well into their adult years. [23]

Women Oppressing Women

Women oppressing women is a broader concept than relational aggression, absent distinctions between indirect, relational, and social aggression. It includes direct (face-to-face) and indirect (behind one's back, where an attacker's identity remains unknown) aggression and all forms of relationally (hurtful words, dirty looks, disparaging sighs, and rolling of eyes) or physically aggressive behavior. Behaviors intended to manipulate, use, or control others are also included, regardless of how such behavior is conveyed.

The *threat* of hurtful behavior (to one's person or threats to damage a relationship) is part of our definition because we consider **any threat of aggression or hurtful behavior as an aggressive**

behavior in its own right, regardless of whether it is conveyed verbally or physically. **A threat of aggression is aggression.**

Hurtful and hostile behaviors may occur at home between mothers, daughters, and sisters; in college or university settings including classes, sororities, or residence halls; in all workplace settings whether women are in the same, lateral, or supervisory positions; and the behaviors cut across all socioeconomic and religious groups, inclusive of all shades of skin, sexual orientation, and social class.

Women Oppressing Women:

is an adult female's injury, harm, or punishment of another woman through or by:

any **verbal or physical threat or act** of aggression, hostility, dominance, subjugation, force, coercion, manipulation, or intimidation used against another woman that harms or intends to harm, hurt, humiliate, embarrass, injure, extort, ruin, or damage a woman's emotional, mental, or physical sense of integrity, well-being, status, reputation, or self-esteem, regardless of the means by which the threat is delivered or action expressed (direct / face-to-face; indirect / covert or circuitous; use of cybertechnology, etc.);

any words or actions that are expressed with the intent to hurt another woman and make her feel bad, undermine her self-esteem, or question her perceptions, sense of self, sense of judgment, or that make her feel she is invisible and does not exist (especially gossip or social exclusion);

any words or actions that use undue emotional pressure or occur with the express intent of withdrawing attention, emotional connection, or affection and that lead to the removal of opportunities for participating in acquaintanceships, friendships, intimate relationships, and social / work groups; or from particular roles, assignments, positions, or activities; or that lead to emotional distance, social exclusion, or social isolation;belittling, condemning, demeaning, devaluing, or lying to another woman out of envy or jealousy of who she is, what she has or represents, or what she might soon achieve or possess;

any use of a computer (e.g., e-mail, instant messaging, text messaging, video), camera phone, cell phone, video camera, recording device, or website as a medium for cyberbullying, with the intent to harm, humiliate, embarrass, injure, extort, or damage another, or her status, reputation, or self-esteem (e.g. embarrassing pictures or videos);

unexpected subtle acts or attitudes experienced by a woman as adverse, such that the act or attitude suggests that she is unworthy and should "stay in her place" (e.g. the only female attorney in a meeting is asked to get coffee for the rest of the male attorneys in the meeting) [Sue, et al., 2007]

encouraging, supporting, or tolerating words or actions that serve to perpetuate the cycle of women oppressing women.

We adapted our definition of women oppressing women from work by Lagerspetz, Bjorkqvist, and Peltonen (1988) and Bjorkqvist (1994) on indirect aggression; Cairns, Cairns, Neckerman, Ferguson, and Gariepy (1989) on social aggression; Crick (1996), Crick and Grotpeter (1995) on relational aggression; and Sue et al., (2007) on microaggressions.

Chapter III

The Female Brain: Wired for Hurt

Women are the focus of gossip and suffer humiliation, betrayal, or social exclusion at the hands of other women with surprising frequency. Hurtful behavior doesn't stop in childhood or adolescence. There are lots of painful memories that stretch through adult life. Regardless of how the hurts occur, the memories of being hurt never fully go away. Consider the possibility that women react differently than a male to betrayal, hurt, and exclusion based on differences in a woman's and man's brain.

Recent neuroscience findings have looked at these differences, including understanding how a woman's brain functions, how social experiences may impact a woman (thus her brain), and how hurtful social experiences (e.g. betrayal, exclusion, gossip) may exact a particular toll on women. Researcher Simon Baron-Cohen, for instance, has highlighted key differences between the male and female brain.[1] Inherent differences between men and women are now better understood given technological advances viewing the brain in the past fifteen years.

Our Social Brain

Countless neuroscientists and authors, such as Daniel Siegel, author of *The Developing Mind* and *The Mindful Brain,* and Allan Schore, author of *Affect Regulation and Repair of the Self,* now describe the brain as the "social organ" of the human body, or as a "relational brain."[2, 3, 4] Along with this changed understanding about brains is a changed view about what has more affect on growth and development—genetic endowment or influences from life experiences.

For a very long time, a debate (the "nature vs. nurture" debate) raged between scientists over this very issue. Most researchers and neuroscientists now agree that the "nature (genetic influence) vs. nurture (influence of experience/environment)" debate is over; they say that "nature and nurture" interact together in an ongoing manner to impact growth and development. Both genetics and experience play important roles, and the interaction between the two is critically important.

All life experiences interact with the brain (biology and genetics, or nature) and mind in a highly interactive manner; first, genetics affect how actual brain structures and the mind develop and function. Life experiences then influence the brain and mind. How a person understands, interprets, and reacts to her life experiences are influenced in return by how the brain and mind function. Lots of trauma, for instance, can affect the normal growth of certain brain structures, and, if this happens, one may not be able to think as clearly or handle feelings as effectively.

Life and social experiences help the brain develop neural pathways or "*wire*" together, starting with the earliest in-utero experiences and continuing throughout life, regardless of the nature of these experiences (from traumatic to difficult to challenging to joyful). Neuroscientists suggest brains are "anticipation machines," so everything a woman experiences at some point in time (even in utero) can become the basis of how she interprets everyday events and experiences. Past experiences, in turn, can affect what she expects to happen in the future and how she interprets future events once they have occurred.

For example, if a young girl felt very criticized and "put-down" by her parents, watched her parents treat each other meanly, was teased and taunted as a child, and was never invited to activities other kids were invited to, then she might think of herself as undesirable and she might feel like an outsider. With this kind of background, it would not be surprising if she anticipated being left out of the same kinds of activities into adolescence or adulthood or began treating others similar to what she watched or experienced in her family. If this same girl grew up in a loving home where she was encouraged and supported in her efforts to grow and she was generally well liked and included in most school and peer activities, then she would likely experience herself as desirable to and comfortable with others as she matured.

Let's go back to Emma and Heather again and the nasty comments made about Heather. Emma had been teased as a child, felt picked on by her older sister, and had watched her parents fight all the time. Emma's family life was marked by hostility and tension, and problems were solved by putting people down. Emma lived what she learned. Because she was accustomed to problems being "solved" in hurtful ways, she repeated these behaviors in her own life. Her brain had "wired up" to experiences of tension and hostility, so she was quick to assume the worst about Heather.

Women's Relational Brains

Digital imaging (MRI and PET scan) and DNA analysis technology have significantly advanced in the past decade and there is now access to information about biological sex differences not previously available in the last century. Scientists have compared the impressions that brains left on the inside of skulls, and these impressions provide insight into how our ancestors lived and thought.[5] These recent science discoveries help describe how female brains have evolved and how these evolutionary changes affect current relationships with other females. Previously, gender differences were believed to be largely based on social and cultural influences that occurred as a child matured into adulthood.

Hormonal Differences: Testosterone, Oxytocin, and Estrogen
Sex hormones have a unique effect on brain organization in the earliest weeks of life, and these hormones affect each child differently depending on the child's biological sex at birth. Dr. Michael Gurian, author of the popular book "*The Wonder of Girls,*"

describes hormonal and brain systems and how they differ between boys and girls. He looked at biochemical and neurobiological research results in approximately thirty cultures. Scientific evidence suggests that every fetal brain begins as a female brain and that the female brain is nature's default brain.[6]

Shortly after conception, changes occur in the fetal brain that significantly affect both the female and male brain. Dr. Louann Brizendine, in her book "*The Female Brain*," describes how at eight weeks after conception a huge testosterone surge occurs (creating male brains) that kills off some cells in the communication centers and grows more cells in the sex and aggression centers. This huge rush of testosterone does not occur in the female brain and as a result the female brain begins to develop further connections in the communication centers and other parts of the brain that process emotion. Dr. Brizendine and others believe that because females have larger communication centers, a female will grow up to be more relationally oriented than males.[7]

Given that females do not experience the testosterone surge in utero that shrinks parts of the brain responsible for communication, processing emotion, and observation, girls end up developing skills in these areas far better than boys. For instance, over the next few years of a girl's life, her eye contact with others and mutual face gazing (key elements of reading and understanding others' emotions) will increase by over 400 percent. Girls are simply born attracted to emotional expression.[8]

Though boys and girls begin to understand who they are based on the interactions they have with others via the "social brain," there are signs early in girls' lives that they more highly value this feedback and likewise are more affected by it. Baby girls rely more heavily on facial signals and cueing from caretakers, and from these interactions girls begin to assess and determine their social worth to others.[9]

Dr. Brizendine suggests females understand the social approval of others at early ages through their ability to comprehend and make meaning out of facial expressions and voice tones. She describes differences even at age one, where boys driven by testosterone will explore, and girls instead will restrain themselves based on both obvious (being told "no") and subtle (facial frown implying "no") social cues to both the girls and boys. Over time, these social cues impact a young girl's sense of herself as successful and important and her understanding of whether or not she is being taken seriously.[10]

Scientists also now have evidence to suggest that as humans were evolving, female relationships were formed to ensure that certain functions vital for survival were carried out. Shelley Taylor, author of "*The Tending Instinct*," researched the stress ("fight or flight") response in females. She suggests that when the stress response is activated in females, the pituitary hormone oxytocin (bonding hormone) is released; oxytocin fosters a response in females to bond with other women and tend to children. When men are faced with danger and their stress response is activated, they will typically fight or flee. Dr. Taylor believes women will find safety, gather and tend to children, and bond with other females for protection when faced with a threat.[11, 12]

As opposed to the "fight or flight" response seen more commonly in men, Taylor described the women's response as "tend and befriend."[13] She notes the tending response is biologically based. Estrogen in women seems to amplify this calming effect, while testosterone seems to reduce it in men. Despite hurtful behavior seen between women, this innate response to stress suggests that females are actually wired to connect and care for each other.

Brain Structure Differences

The Hippocampus and Memory

The hippocampus is principally responsible for forming and storing long-term memory. Dr. Gurian notes that females have a larger hippocampus than males. In the hippocampus itself, the female brain produces steady connections with memories of intimate details. Gurian suggests this structural difference may have evolved because females needed to care for their young as well as gather and forage food. Consequently structures such as the hippocampus may have helped females remember details to aid in the survival of their young.[14] Perhaps this information can also help explain why females are more likely to remember details of people's lives, whether the details are used for bonding and promoting connections with others or for hurting them.

Dr. David Geary, a professor at the University of Missouri, noted that male brains contain about 6.5 times more gray matter, sometimes called "thinking matter" than compared to women. Female brains, by contrast, have more than 9.5 times as much white matter than male brains. White matter is responsible for connecting together various parts of the brain. Differences between gray and white matter in men and women help explain why females have more dominant language skills when compared to men. Geary suggests that women use these skills to their advantage by using language more when they compete, including using language to gossip and manipulate information. Gossiping and manipulative behavior (relational aggression) may have given females a survival advantage long ago.[15]

Olivia, a co-worker of mine (Erika), told me that she recently interviewed a friend of many years for a position in her agency. While her friend had many good qualifications, she did not have the proper credentials to fill the position. Olivia used much discretion as she told her friend that she was not selected for the follow-up interview and employment. A few days later, Olivia received a spiteful message on her cell phone calling Olivia malicious names and belittling her using details of their earlier shared experiences, to the point that Olivia was in tears by the time the message ended. Olivia knew it was the woman she interviewed. She was deeply affected by her hurtful words and described feeling miserable for days as she replayed in her mind all the cruel remarks that were made.

Given women's relational brains and ability to remember details with accuracy, perhaps women are also more deeply hurt by actions that betray, backstab, trash-talk, or exclude.

Language

Most women find biological comfort in one another's company, and language is felt as the glue that bonds females together. Girls begin to talk earlier than boys; some verbal areas of the brain are larger in females than in males.[16] The female corpus collosum is about 25 percent bigger than a male's by about seventeen years of age, which provides women with the ability to "cross talk" (share information) between the hemispheres of their brains; one result of such "cross-talk" is the ability to verbalize emotions more efficiently.[17]

Deborah Tannen's best-seller "*You Just Don't Understand: Women and Men in Conversation*" claims that while men use conversation "to preserve their independence and negotiate and maintain status in a hierarchical social order," women use conversation as "a way of establishing connections and negotiating relationships."[18] There are some differences in the languages of men and women, and Tannen suggests that men respond to problems with concrete solutions and suggestions and women respond with empathy and an emphasis on community. She identified female talk as "rapport talk" and male talk as "report talk."[19] One key reason for this difference is that females have 15 percent more blood flow in their brains with more energy flowing to more areas in the female brain, which means that the female brain may feel like it never shuts down. A female brain is continuously craving increased bonding, attachment, and close stimulation because intimate stimulation is what gives females pleasure.[20]

Dr. Brizendine also believes there is a biological reason that females connect through talking and sharing secrets with one another. Connecting through talking activates certain areas of the brain that respond to pleasure. When females connect and talk to each other they receive a large neurological reward. Dopamine and oxytocin (brain chemicals) are released; they trigger feelings of intimacy and stimulate the motivation and pleasure circuits in the brain. The pleasurable feelings further reinforce the desire to connect and bond and result in a sense of harmony and well-being.[21]

⊲✣⊳

Empathic Responsivity

Carol Gilligan, in her groundbreaking book "*In a Different Voice*," noted that male group behavior is characterized by an emphasis on space, privacy, and autonomy, and female group behavior by a need to feel included, connected, and attached.[22] Much later, Simon Baron-Cohen in his book "*The Essential Difference*" suggested the female brain is hard-wired for empathy while the male brain is predominantly hard-wired for understanding and building systems.[23]

Baron-Cohen notes that baby girls as young as one year old respond more empathically than boys to the pain of other people, showing greater concern by displaying sad looks, soothing sounds, and reassurance. This responsivity is seen in women too, with more women reporting spending time soothing others. Baron-Cohen notes women are also more sensitive to facial expressions and are better at decoding non-verbal communication and judging a person's character. Brizendine agrees, stating that from day one, baby girls are designed to pick up and process subtle emotional cues that confirm their worthiness and lovability and that also build empathy skills.[24, 25]

Anne Campbell, author of *A Mind of Her Own: The Evolutionary Psychology of Women,* also notes that women are better than men at reading and responding to subtle cues about mood and temperament. Females are also more trusting of others, more empathic, and more focused on one-on-one friendships. Human and primate studies suggest that friendship does for females what status does for males; female bonding enhances a sense of well-being while also improving an offspring's prospects for survival.[26, 27]

Specific structural and hormonal differences between the male and female brain have been identified through scientific research. Differences include a female's ability to attend to social cues, remember details better, desire social connection and bonding/closeness, use language, and communicate more effectively than men. From an evolutionary standpoint, overall it appears a female grows up to be more relationally oriented than males.

These differences may have played a key role in how women's brains have changed and evolved over time. Since females had to play it safe and ensure they were not physically hurt, they learned to aggress in different ways than men. Perhaps relational aggression is hard-wired into female human consciousness. Women could not risk direct or physical aggression due to children being physically dependent on their survival. So women learned to use their words and other manipulative actions to hurt one another.

The Pain of Social Exclusion

Louann Brizendine suggests the female brain has a stronger reaction to relationship conflict and rejection than does the male brain. Men can take pleasure in interpersonal quarrels and competition; they even get a positive boost from it. However, in women, conflict can release a surge of negative chemical reactions, creating feelings of stress, upset, and dread. Even if a woman thinks that there might be an impending conflict, it will be read by the female brain as threatening the relationship, thus evoking unpleasant feelings within her.[28] Let's follow her thinking.

A woman starts feeling anxious, cut-off, and fearful of being rejected and alone when a relationship is threatened or lost, and this is a time when the stress hormone cortisol predominates. At the risk of conflict or threats to relationship, other neurotransmitters such as serotonin, dopamine, and oxytocin (the bonding hormone) decrease dramatically. Understand that a woman derives feelings of closeness from the flow of oxytocin, which is boosted by the social contact she has with others. But the minute that social contact is gone and the oxytocin and dopamine significantly decrease, she may feel headed for emotional trouble.[29]

Modern medical imaging techniques have demonstrated that the pain of social exclusion arises in part from the same brain regions that report physical pain; in animal experiments, opioid pain reducers like morphine, and increased levels of the brain's own pain-blocking endorphins, also blunted the pain of social loss. Jaak Panksepp, author of *Affective Neuroscience: The Foundations of Human and Animal Emotions*, notes that psychological pain in humans, especially grief and intense loneliness, may in fact share some of the same neural pathways that are seen when someone is experiencing physical pain. The reason appears to be survival. Emotional (and physical) pain hurts. So humans have a desire and natural inclination to move closer to others to relieve the pain.[30]

Francine Shapiro, in the book *Healing Trauma: Attachment, Mind, Body and Brain*, describes why the effects of social exclusion, a type of trauma, may be so profound. Shapiro considers *trauma* any negative event that has had a lasting effect upon the self or psyche.[31] Not only can a trauma include having experienced or witnessed tragic life experiences, it can include lesser incidents of humiliation, conflict, rejection, or emotional neglect. She suggests that even early childhood experiences of humiliations, conflicts, and rejections can have a lasting effect on a person's psyche because these exclusionary experiences act as the "evolutionary equivalent of being cut out of the herd."[32]

Just imagine how many times girls and women are excluded from groups and activities. Imagine, too, the feelings from being excluded . . . feelings of anger, disappointment, sadness, embarrassment, shame, and a sense of being defective. Rachel Simmons, author of *Odd Girl Out*, notes that girls find the fear of solitude overpowering and that they "may try to avoid being alone at all costs."[33] No doubt repeated experiences of being excluded could erode a woman's sense of self.

Think, too, about what happens when women treat each other hurtfully. If you recall your own experiences of humiliation or rejection, you can understand why these experiences seem so intense. Not only is there pain of being embarrassed or socially excluded, the exclusion itself can leave a woman feeling she is faced with the threat of being left to survive all alone —left out and wandering in an "emotional wilderness," which results in even more feelings—those of anxiety and fear.

Nora, mother of twelve-year-old twins Jessica and Julie, attended one of our talks. Nora explained that recently she noticed important behavior differences between her girls. Both of the twins have bright red hair and freckles and are the butt of much teasing. For unknown reasons, they have been left out of many activities with their peers. Julie, however, reacted differently than her sister to teasing and being left out. Julie shut down, retreated to the safety of her room, and became depressed; Jessica made efforts to brush it aside and develop a different group of friends.

Research shows that when a child or adolescent is teased or harassed, cortisol levels (indicating the level of stress) rise in her brain. When these levels of cortisol continue to rise for a prolonged period of time, other brain and hormonal activity will decrease or even stop completely. If she continues to be picked on without any intervention, her brain will be considerably affected and she will "rewire" neurologically. Girls who experience this type of abuse often become quiet, withdrawn, have difficulty eating and trouble communicating.[34] When girls don't receive positive emotional connections they desire and need they can become extremely depressed and withdrawn. The hurt and pain from damaged or ruptured connections is real, as is the fear of being left all alone to survive the pain.

One reason women may choose to relate more with men is because of the hurt women feel when betrayed or excluded by their female friends; it just becomes too painful to experience. Since females are wired to be relational, perhaps betrayal by women feels even more painful.

Roots of Female Competition and Aggression

Many people have asked whether women hurting women is really a new phenomenon. Scientific discoveries about human evolution suggest the answer is no. Evolutionary psychologists, such as Anne Campbell, author of *A Mind of Her Own,* believe that female-to-female aggression actually has roots in early human behavior.[35, 36]

Physical Size

The most obvious view, that women use less physical and less dangerous forms of aggression on the basis of size differences between men and women, offers only an initial explanation of relational aggression.

Survival and Tending to the Children

Historically, infants have been more dependent on mothers than fathers for survival. Women were responsible for child care during pregnancy, breast feeding, and generally throughout most of childhood and adolescence. Consequently, if a mother wanted her child to survive, she had to be continuously concerned with her own survival as well.

Because a woman had to be so concerned with and careful about her own and her children's survival, females collectively evolved to care more about danger than males. Women learned to use low-risk and indirect, as opposed to more direct, stereotypically male forms of aggression (physical force and pain) to successfully survive. Using less dangerous aggressive behavior helped protect women from getting hurt and helped ensure literal physical survival for conceiving and tending to children. Women learned to compete with other women without risking their lives, and instead behaved aggressively by ostracizing, stigmatizing, and excluding others socially. In this manner, a woman could still be aggressive without having to engage in direct physical confrontations.[37]

Competing for Resources: Men, Reproductive Success, and Status

Anne Campbell suggests females compete with one another to enhance reproductive success and gain resources that can subsequently be passed to their children; males compete with one another for status and to gain power and resources because these are assets that may improve their reproductive success.[38] From an evolutionary standpoint, aggression between males can be seen as potentially beneficial; it allows aggressive males to produce more offspring and similarly allows them to genetically pass on aggressive characteristics to their male offspring,—elements that help ensure survival.[39]

Competition between women based on beauty and physical attractiveness is common. Perhaps you have felt those pressures yourself. There are evolutionary pressures at play here. Campbell explains that men place a greater premium upon physical attractiveness than do women; for males, one of the primary criteria for mate selection is attractiveness, as defined by a youthful body and face.[40]

Women go to exhausting lengths to achieve a youthful, beautiful appearance to effectively compete with other women. Look at the multi-billion dollar marketing efforts, beauty products, and now TV shows (*Dr. 90210, 10 Years Younger, The Swan*) directed at helping women maintain a youthful appearance and the significance of this competition comes clear.

It's easy to identify the countless arenas in which this competition takes place: being a cheerleader or pep squad member, being selected into a sorority, modeling, acting, or broadcasting. It is a well-known fact that attractive people are hired more quickly and more often than less attractive people, and that attractive people often make more money. The list of benefits for those who are attractive is quite long.

The downside is that attractiveness sometimes incites jealousy in other women, which, at times, has resulted in hurtful behavior and violence between women. Anne Campbell suggests that females may also compete with each other for access to high-quality males using *both* physical and indirect aggression. Examples of such behavior have clearly been promoted and seen on reality TV shows such as *Age of Love, The Bachelor,* and *Flavor of Love.* Women can be seen spitting on, tearing at the hair of, shoving, and hitting other women.

From an evolutionary perspective, women will use hostile, hurtful, and other relationally aggressive behaviors against other women based on physical size, personal and child survival needs, and to compete for resources, which include a man who can ensure reproductive success and other resources such as status and power.

Women have an intense desire to relate and connect, yet they experience emotional and physical stress from conflict or the threat of conflict. The brain experiences emotional pain and physical pain similarly. Potential or actual exclusion from desired groups and cliques can be experienced as the evolutionary equivalent of being left to survive all alone. Perhaps the "wiring" of the "very" relational female brain intensifies effects of hurtful and hostile behavior experienced by women. Instead of bonding and emotional closeness, there is pain.

Chapter IV

Catfight! How the Media Portrays
and Trivializes Women

I (Erika) had just attended the annual American Psychological Association Convention and while at the airport waiting for my flight back home, I picked up a US Weekly magazine (August 27, 2007) just before boarding my plane. I knew there would be news of some female celebrity pitted against her "female rival." The ninth page headline read "The Hills Feud Gets Worse!", and without fail the page was split with the two women positioned back-to-back. The article focus: "Will the Hills' catfights ever end?"

Magazines have frequently used "catfighting" headlines to increase sales by highlighting female-to-female hostility and betrayal. Magazine racks and airwaves remain saturated with stories of female rivals. A sampling of the check-out aisle in any grocery store carried these cover headlines: *US Weekly* magazine read "Denise Steals Heather's Husband"; next to it the *Star* read "Victim or Vixen" with a picture of Denise Richard in the middle of Heather Locklear and Charlie Sheen. During that same month another cover of *US Weekly* declared "Fight! Boy Trouble! Lindsay makes Jessica cry in public as a screaming match turns violent." There is the well-known feud between Nicole Ritchie and Paris Hilton … just one more example of media-driven conflict and hostility between women.

Mass media (e.g. television, movies, computer/Internet, print, and advertising) reflects where we are as a society and it also influences where we may be headed. It acts as a force for socializing women, often one that supports and fosters a culture of women's hostility toward other women. Traditional stereotypes of women are maintained regardless of media venue. Female competition is positioned and marketed, and images of women fighting and being hostile to one another have increased. The messages are predictable and enduring.

Media is more than mere entertainment. It teaches, persuades, and shapes lives, offering guidelines about who women should be, how to behave, and how to interact with others. Media portrayal of women is often devaluing. Women are compared negatively to other women, portrayed as marginally powerful or objectified sexually; these are the messages women so frequently internalize. Rarely is legitimate competition and valid anger portrayed between women. Mostly it is trivialized or it is not taken seriously.

Women and Television

Between us (Erika and Joan), we grew up across the '60s, '70s, '80s, and '90s, years filled with watching a countless array of television shows (e.g. *The Cosby Show, The Wonder Years, Roseanne, Friends, Will and Grace . . .* or digging back farther . . . *That Girl, Leave it to Beaver, The Dick Van Dyke Show, Father Knows Best, I Love Lucy*), which were more focused on family, community, and communication. Though some of the early programs sugar-coated or avoided addressing difficult life situations, or resolved the plot issue by the end of the program, underneath it all, humor and sarcasm included, the bottom line message was one of emphasizing relationship connections or family bonds, friends, or community. Television programming today, however, seems to predominantly highlight the things that expose, humiliate, hurt, or divide women. Hostility, deception, and conflict are emphasized instead.

Situation comedies or solid dramas that were once the norm have been largely replaced by reality TV shows. With "reality television" it's difficult to tell how much of the content is in fact reality based or instead contrived to make "good TV." Many of these reality based programs focus on young women, typically between the ages of eighteen and twenty-nine, and the women are usually portrayed negatively. Women hurting or betraying other women (*Gossip Girl, Bad Girl's Club*) is marketed and sensationalized.

Consider TV headlines and images that involve women fighting against each other. *The Bachelor* promo announces "The backstabbing begins!" For *Joe Millionaire* it was: "The claws come out" and "girls can be conniving, deceiving, and vicious." One contestant brags, "I know better than to trust women." Tyra declared just before she eliminated a contestant on *America's Next Top Model*, "One thing with your intelligence is that it can intimidate people." Tyra's remark is a great example of one double bind that women experience, that of having a brain and a womb, yet being viewed as not being able to use both simultaneously.

Other recent examples of highly rated TV programs that positioned women against each other include *The Apprentice*, *The Bachelor*, *America's Next Top Model*, *Elimidate*, *The Hills*, *Gossip Girl*, and the *Bad Girls Club*. Whether the reality TV programs are real or fake, they continue to marginalize, stereotype, and oppress women and influence social and cultural norms, making quite acceptable hostile and hateful treatment of each other.

Looking for "The Money Shot": Women and TV Ratings

Reality TV shows make efforts to produce "*The Money Shot*." *The Money Shot* is film slang for scene(s) that can significantly boost TV ratings; a high show rating translates into more money for a TV show. Producers, directors, and editors all know that one of the best *"money shots"*, one that creates a lot of "buzz" for a show, high ratings, and good money, is when women (especially young, attractive, and sexy women) humiliate themselves or each other to win a prize; verbally or physically fight against each other to get a man; or engage in deceit or trickery to win a competition.

One of the latest shows in the string of reality based TV programs that highlight women hurting, betraying, or backstabbing other women was dubbed Age of Love. The advertisement for the show highlighted the "Cougars vs. Kittens" and the narrator promised that "the claws will come out" as "each week, you'll see young versus old in a battle for love." The forty- year-old "Cougars" were competing against the twenty-year-old "Kittens" for the affections of a thirty-year-old tennis star named Mark. The network called the show a "social experiment" and asked "does age really matter when it comes to love?" The program used the same basic premise as many other reality shows— women compete against one another with some women portrayed as "good" and some as "evil" . . . and some women always getting hurt. When the twenty-something "kittens" are first introduced, they are exhibited provocatively in a descending glass elevator. Later they are shown in their apartment "hula hooping" while the "cougars" are shown in their apartment quietly doing needlepoint and laundry.

Consider the social messages embedded in these images. The messages emphasize youth, attractiveness, and sexuality . . . used all for the pursuit of a man. No effort is made to address intelligence, ambition, warmth, good character, and pursuit of the woman's goals for herself, the very elements that strengthen a woman's positive experience of herself. Women in their twenties are sent the message to accentuate and highlight sexuality, while females in their forties appear to have lost their sexuality and perhaps also their intelligence; instead they are left focusing their energy on domestic activities. Not only did this show perpetuate negative stereotypes about young and older women, the central focus of the show was the competition between these groups of women as they fought each other for a man.

The show became less focused on "competition" and more focused on bringing women down. As women were eliminated from the show and the two groups of women began sharing a house together, they were portrayed as more vicious and nasty toward each other. The sad reality is that these images negatively affect our legitimacy as women having much more to offer than our sexuality and much more to achieve than getting a date.

Media Images of Women

There is a saying that the more something changes, the more it stays the same. This cliché fits how various types of media treat girls and women. While there are many more depictions of women in movies and TV who have central roles, character strength, wisdom, and leadership positions, there are a greater number that denigrate women and place them in roles where they are hostile to other women.

Women are inundated with information on a daily basis and the sheer number of images from which to choose is overwhelming. Images displayed by virtually every media venue socialize women into their proper place; model hostile, deceptive, and destructive behaviors between women; and offer fewer opportunities for women to emulate positive role models or make sense of what they view and experience. It is no wonder that women turn against each other.

Stereotypes of women are packaged through all venues, from television (regular programming and commercials), film, radio, music lyrics, websites, and Internet advertising to billboards to t-shirts. Anywhere something can be marketed, such packaging occurs. Consider how the media directed attention to superficial aspects of women. In July 2007, presidential candidate Senator Hillary Clinton was talking on television about the cost of higher education. Media focus quickly turned to Clinton's pink jacket, black shirt with a slight v-neck, and, what is evident at closer scrutiny, a shadowy bit of cleavage, as opposed to the serious topic content. For the next couple days, news outlets and websites were mired in reporting only about Hillary's cleavage.

This media situation is an example of a double bind. Women can either have a womb and be sexual or have a brain. Any hint of sexuality and the intellectual discussion gets lost. Women are socialized to be sexy, but admonished simultaneously for using sexuality to attract attention or advance their careers. Equally as confusing . . . many female reporters were neither redirecting the conversation nor defending Hillary.

The New Disney for Adult Women

In presentations and workshops, I (Erika) talk about familiar media images of women who hurt and deceive each other. Disney princess characters . . . Ariel from *The Little Mermaid*, Belle from *Beauty and the Beast*, and Jasmine from *Aladdin* offer places to start. These images are well-known to most women; as little girls they were showered with Disney princess pictures, toys, and clothes.

Disney films have socialized most girls, so it's worth taking a deeper look into the "Disney spell." You are already quite familiar with the story of Cinderella and how she competed with her cruel, backstabbing, "evil" stepsisters to win the heart of the prince. Now consider the parallel between another popular Disney film and one similarly popular dating reality show.

Disney brought us the story of Ariel, a sixteen-year-old mermaid who gives up her voice in exchange for legs to be with a prince. Ursula, a sea witch, convinces Ariel that on land it's more appropriate for women to remain silent, and Ariel agrees to the deal offered by Ursula. If Ariel fails to get a kiss from the prince within three days, then Ariel must give up her soul to the evil witch Ursula. Ariel learns that the prince is already engaged to another woman and is heartbroken. In the end, Ariel does win the prince, but not until Ursula tries to kill Ariel. Ultimately Ursula gets killed by the prince.

In a very obvious way, the film models intentional and purposeful betrayal between women and the silencing of the female voice (one through a deal, the other through death). A woman who trusts other women may find trusting women a situation potentially fraught with danger; women can "take away souls." The only thing worth selling your "soul" for is a man.

With highlights of the Little Mermaid in mind, consider the contestants seen on the popular American dating reality series *The Bachelor* (2002), where twenty-five contestants compete for the heart of one man. Every episode ends with "the bachelor" eliminating women from the show. It has been a ratings hit since its debut and there have been several spin-offs.

So what is the parallel between Ariel and the women on the bachelor program? Think about it . . . a little girl learns at two, three, six, or ten years of age that she must give up a part of herself, compete with other girls to get a boy, and that it is hard to trust relationships with other girls. As girls mature, they learn that it is okay to make "deals with the devil," to give up parts of themselves (particularly their voices), and that they may have to scheme to get a boy or a man, all at the expense of themselves and other girls/women. These expectations, norms, and values get internalized, and women often believe these views and behaviors are normal.

The women on *The Bachelor* series are similar in the sense that they scheme and lie to make each other look bad so that they won't be eliminated from the show. They gossip about each other to intentionally hurt one another and essentially give up parts of themselves to be with the "prince," who they barely even know. Do they really want to be with this man or is it that they have internalized messages from our culture that women are "supposed" to compete with each other to win the heart of a prince? Is there really any difference between parts of the film in *The Little Mermaid* and the theme of *The Bachelor?*

Images of Women: Socialized to New Lows

If you are familiar with recent television shows, there are scenes from the "reality" dating show *Elimidate,* where one participant chooses between four contestants of the opposite sex for a date, eliminating them one by one. Female contestants "confessed" to strong feelings of competition; they leveled insults or physically fought in many episodes and scenes. It was more a show about a nasty competition between women rather than dating, as most shows highlighted the arguing, bickering, and physical fights for the prize . . . a man. A frequently viewed video clip (found on YouTube.com) from the 2006 and 2007 ratings hit *Flavor of Love*, a "dating reality show" with a similar format, shows two women spewing hateful words, spitting, and on the verge of a physical fight. In a spin-off from this show, producers promised viewers *"Hair may be pulled. Spit may fly. Fists may land. But one thing is for sure, when these ladies stab each other in the back— it will be with the proper utensil."* Or there is *The Apprentice*, which also featured women hurting women. In Season I, contestants Omarosa Manigault-Stallworth and Ereka Vetrini and their "catfights" were highlighted. Omarosa accused Ereka of calling her a racial slur and the show played up this tension as a featured storyline between the women throughout several episodes.

Sunset Tan (2007) is another reality show that showcased women being mean to and competing against one another. The focus of this E! Television network show is about the lives of the managers and employees of the Sunset Tan tanning salon in Los Angeles and the competition between them to be selected as the manger of the new Las Vegas salon. With the exception of one brunette, all of the young women closely resemble each other (long, bleached blonde hair, tall, pretty, and tan). Think about young girls watching this show. They are socialized to emulate young women who are cruel to one another as they compete for employment at a tanning salon in Las Vegas.

Or consider a TV advertisement that was broadcast to millions of viewers during the 2002 Superbowl football game. It is another illustration of how the media portrays women hurting women. Miller Lite ran a beer ad entitled "Catfight," which portrayed two beautiful women turning the classic Miller Lite debate of "tastes great—less filling" into a brawl. In front of predominantly male spectators who are part of the actual ad, the two women get into an angry argument, ripping each other's clothes off and end up in panties and bras wrestling in mud.

What can be drawn from this ad? The ad denigrates women and suggests it is totally appropriate to solve problems and resolve disputes through physical fights. The fight itself is sexualized, so violence and sexuality get paired as being okay, and since men do nothing to break up the fight and are enjoying it, the fight between women is not taken seriously and is instead nothing more than a spectator sport. It seems only to be a small leap for women as a group to not be taken seriously . . . and then for a woman not to take herself seriously.

The unrelenting images of women competing for a man's affection have been matched by the degree of hostility and betrayal between women conveyed on screen. Now there are more images of women who behave as uncaring persons and who exhibit disrespectful, mean, deceptive, and cruel behavior toward each other. The more these images are conveyed, the more acceptable they become and the more children are socialized to use these behaviors to relate with one another for solving problems between them. How much worse will it get? To what degree will we allow our everyday behavior to deteriorate if we continue to tolerate less and less humane and loving treatment of each other?

On July 11, 2008, the N Network, a channel targeted specifically to a teen audience, premiered its new reality series called *Queen Bees*. The eight-episode series took an inside look at seven self-absorbed, narcissistic "mean girls," who were nominated to be on the show by family members, boyfriends, and friends in the hope that they will have a serious change of heart . . . and behavior. While the girls think they are competing to be the biggest diva in the house, they quickly learn they are there because people want them to change. Each young girl is asked to re-examine her hurtful demeanor. The incentive? The girl that changes and becomes the nicest wins $25,000. It seems there are positive aspects to this show given that the focus is intended to address today's "mean girls" problem. Here is a show, offering money as incentive, where girls compete against one another to improve their attitudes and behavior to that of civility and human decency. Can a girl really change her mean behavior in just eight episodes?

Certainly, the show's intent is headed in the right direction, yet there is deeper hurt and anger experienced by girls who inflict pain on another girl. No television show can really get to the root of this pain in just eight episodes. Yet it begs the question . . . how did we get here in the first place? What changed culturally that we have supported and been desensitized to such hurtful behavior between girls or between women?

Despite how obviously these shows exploit and demean women, we have heard men say that they love these types of shows because they think it is sexy to watch women compete and fight with one another. Besides the romantic nature of the shows, some women say they love these shows because they feel stronger and more powerful; watching some women fail and demoralize each other somehow makes other women feel better about themselves. What is difficult here, of course, is that the women watching the shows do not yet fully understand how they are like the women on the show; when any woman is treated in such a demoralizing manner, it devalues all women.

Social Pressures Take Their Toll

A 2007 American Psychological Association Task Force on how media affects young children reported that children under the age of eight are unable to critically comprehend televised advertising messages and are prone to accept advertiser messages as truthful, accurate, and unbiased.[1] When girls watch these "reality" TV shows and watch women compete in a hostile manner, hurt, and betray each other then their perceptions of reality can become altered enough to believe that this is how women should act and behave. Advertising, TV, and movies strongly influence how girls treat each other, and these media images often create a climate between girls and women that is hostile and damaging. When girls fully absorb and imitate these negative behaviors, it may be more difficult for them to form solid friendships and close emotional bonds with each other.

As clinicians, we work with many female adolescents who have been subjected to negative media portrayal of girls and women. Look at how the effects of the media played out in real life with one young girl.

I (Erika) recently worked as the therapist for a thirteen-year-old girl who made a serious suicide attempt by overdosing on sleeping pills. She had been referred to me for talking back to teachers and her parents, physically fighting with girls, and for engaging in promiscuous behaviors. When I met Kaylee, she had just turned thirteen and I was struck by her appearance. She was heavily made up, had long, dark hair, and was wearing very short shorts and a low-cut top. Kaylee was thirteen going on thirty. Initially Kaylee had difficulty opening up to me and I felt like I was pulling teeth just to get her to talk about how she was feeling. After several sessions, Kaylee began to tell me how she felt pressured and "worn out." The demands on her as a young girl felt hard and unrelenting; she was trying to do well in school, to be pretty, and to be liked by her peers.

She believed she was inadequate and worthless, and felt like she could never live up to what she saw on TV or from the posts she found on MySpace and YouTube. The pressures to have sex, to use sex to get attention, or to try to be stunningly attractive so she could be accepted and seen as desirable to boys in school were all overwhelming. She said she frequently watched shows like *Girl's Behaving Badly*, a show that lives up to its name by how it plays up hostile competition between the girls. Kaylee felt like she had to compete with her friends to get boys' attention. Kaylee wanted so badly to be liked, yet she ended up physically attacking another thirteen-year-old girl because the other girl was gossiping about Kaylee's sexual behavior. Gossiping by the other girls hurt her more than anything she had ever experienced. Once Kaylee was doing much better, we ended therapy. A few months later I learned that Kaylee was in the hospital for seriously slashing her wrists. Kaylee's mom told me that it was prompted by the girls in school digitally cropping a sexualized picture of her and passing it around on the school campus.

We see many girls and women just like Kaylee, who feel strong social pressure to behave a particular way or to live up to a certain image and they don't just feel these pressures from their peers. They are constantly bombarded with messages to compete with each other for a man, for a job, for status, prestige, or for some other prize, and clearly they internalize these messages. These issues, however, are less commonly discussed; one consequence is that girls and women do not learn how to critically evaluate the messages they see and hear, nor do they learn how to effectively cope with such intense competition and overwhelming pressure.

The "Packaging" of Girls and Women Through Advertising

Statistics compiled by TV Free America suggest that the television is turned on for almost seven hours each day in the average American household, and the average American watches more than four hours each day. Girls consume approximately thirty-eight hours of television per week and women watch nearly six hours of television per day (an hour more than men!). The average television viewer will see ninety-five to one hundred commercials per day, paying closer attention to roughly sixty of them. Researchers estimate that an average child sees 360,000 advertisements on TV by the time she reaches age eighteen.[2] Large corporations generally spend several hundreds of millions of dollars annually on magazine advertising alone; a typical magazine reader will have seen sixty-five to seventy print ads in one day.

We interviewed Dr. Jean Kilbourne for our *Women's Inspiration* radio show about media images of women. She is a noted expert on the use of women and men in advertising and she described how girls and women are continuously objectified in the media.[3] Dr. Kilbourne noted that advertising is over a $200 billion a year industry and that across all media females are exposed to over 3,000 ads a day. Despite being bombarded by all these media messages, girls and women commonly believe they are not influenced by advertising. Our conversations with many girls and women support this view. They believe they are not influenced when the media portrays women hurting, betraying, and backstabbing each other. They remain quite unaware of how much these images hurt women and keep them oppressed. Yet girls do resort to indirect ways of handling their competitive and aggressive feelings based on what they see in the media.

A study by Emily Hamilton, Laurie Mintz, and Susan Kabushek-West verified that a woman's dissatisfaction with her own body image worsened after viewing magazine advertisement images of women who exemplified cultural standards of the thin beauty ideal.[4] If dissatisfaction occurred after only a brief viewing of magazine advertisements, just think of the overall effect of repeated viewing from all sources of media and what continuous exposure might do to a girl's and a woman's self-image and behavior.

Marketing tactics have changed and advertisements now use highly sexualized images of young girls. Drs. Sharon Lamb and Lyn Mikel Brown, in their book *Packaging Girlhood,* have written extensively about marketing and media influences on girls. They outline for parents the image of girls that is packaged and sold to their daughters, and how a girl's personal power and sense of self has been co-opted by marketers of music, fashion, books, cartoons, TV shows, movies, toys, and more. Girls are "packaged" for consumption and then "sold" how to behave.[5]

Girls today are socialized at much earlier ages than their mothers and grandmothers to behave, dress, and relate to others in a more sexualized manner. Consistent media messages delivered to young girls and women emphasize being seen as beautiful, confident, thin, happy, and sexual. As a reflection of these changing social values, I (Erika) opened up a recent Sunday edition of the *Los Angeles Times* newspaper to find the Target store mailer advertising girls clothing that I mistook for women's clothes! The girls in the pictures appeared to be around eight years old, yet they were dressed in sexy, tight clothing as if they were featured in a Victoria's Secret catalogue.

M. Gigi Durham also tackles the issue of media influences on girls in her book *The Lolita Effect: The Media Sexualization of Young Girls and What We Can Do About It*. She contends that the media propagate a narrowly defined, and thus damaging, version of female sexuality such that it hinders a girl's healthy development and sense of self-empowerment. She notes that the current sexualization of young girls is an outgrowth of many cultural factors; it includes corporate media that eroticize childhood for profit. She describes five core myths of sexuality circulated by mainstream media with children and adolescents as their target audience.[6] They include:

Five Core Myths of Sexuality

1) [myth of] the "perfect body" – slender, yet curvy and preferably Caucasian
2) flaunting such a body is the only way to express sexuality and femininity
3) girls need to please and attract boys, but their own pleasure is inconsequential
4) the younger the girl is, the sexier she is
5) violence is sexy

(Durham, 2008)

Drs. Diane Levin and Jean Kilbourne also discuss these ideas in their book, *So Sexy, So Soon: The New Sexualized Childhood and What Parents Can Do to Protect Their Kid.* Girls are exposed to messages that they can't just be girls; they must grow up faster and faster, and this pressure can have far-reaching and potentially devastating consequences.

Though girls' and women's bodies are being used to sell, the latest implications of using sexuality are quite serious. Dr. Kilbourne poignantly described how sexuality is being used to socialize all of us to develop relationships to products as opposed to authentic and enduring relationships with each other.[7]

Women are clearly influenced by the barrage of images. The loss of personal power, poor sense of self and resulting self-hatred is the basis of hurtful behavior. Remember, Kaylee (Erika's client) attempted suicide as a result of too much pressure to look, act, and behave a particular way; the pressures became too overwhelming for her. Many women resort to taking out their anger and aggression on themselves, as Kaylee did, or each other, because the pressures to be a certain way are too difficult to bear.

In 2007, the American Psychological Association's Task Force on the Sexualization of Girls concluded that the sexualization of girls is a broad and increasing problem and is harmful to girls' self-image and healthy development (see text box). Examples of sexualization are found in all forms of media, and as "new media" have been created and access to media has become omnipresent, examples of harmful behavior have increased.[8] Websites designed for the sole purpose of degrading and humiliating women can also be found. Likewise, the Internet, via e-mail, chat rooms, or social networking sites, is used as a weapon of "miss destruction."

The APA Task Force Report

Sexualization has negative effects on:

Cognitive and emotional health:

Sexualization and objectification undermine a person's confidence in and comfort with her own body, leading to emotional and self-image problems, such as shame and anxiety.

Mental and physical health:

Research links sexualization with three of the most common mental health problems diagnosed in girls and women— eating disorders, low self-esteem, and depression or depressed mood.

Sexual development:

Research suggests that the sexualization of girls has negative consequences on girls' ability to develop a healthy sexual self-image.

When only a few people talk about how the media socializes girls and women into stereotyped roles and hostile behavior, or how women oppressing women is sensationalized on TV, then girls and women anticipate their reality will be similar to what they watch. Dr. George Gerbner and his colleagues suggested that television is responsible for shaping or cultivating viewers' ideas of their own social world, and that the television world is not a window on or reflection of the world, but a world in itself. When a viewer believes that what she is watching on TV is real, then her reality becomes grossly altered.[9] The more one watches television and is exposed to distortions of reality without questioning the assumptions and intention behind the programming, the more that person will view the real world as similar to the world portrayed on television.

Something to Think About

Pay close attention to messages you receive as you watch TV, listen to music, surf the Internet, or see magazine covers that position women against each other. How do these images affect you and your relationships with other females? How do they affect your relationships with males? Think about ways you can help change how several media sources negatively portray female relationships.

Take action: turn off the TV, write to producers and editors to change storylines that promote positive images of female-to-female relationships, or speak out and voice your thoughts about programming in your own community. Become *media literate*— knowledgeable about the media's impact on your behavior. See information and questions in Appendix B.

Chapter V

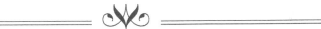

Damned if You Do,
Damned if You Don't

Women are often encouraged to assert themselves—to speak or stand up for their needs and rights. Sounds reasonable and seems like a logical message to follow. However, a woman also hears the message that if she does assert herself, then she could be characterized as "bitchy" or "more like a man."

Like the example above, a woman experiences a variety of mixed messages as she matures, and these mixed messages influence her sense of identity. You may best know them as a "*Catch-22*," a phrase taken from Joseph Heller's book by the same name.[1] The *Catch-22* is described as: a circumstance that denies a solution; an illogical, unreasonable, or senseless situation; a situation presenting two equally undesirable alternatives; or a hidden difficulty or means of entrapment.[2] For instance, a woman is encouraged to be attractive and sexy, but if she dresses too provocatively, she might be called a slut.

Gregory Bateson described a mixed message as a *double bind* in 1972.[3] He said a *double bind* occurs when contradictory demands are made on an individual, so that no matter which demand is followed, the individual's response will be construed as incorrect. Double binds are also known as *"no-win"* situations.

When any kind of message is repeated enough times, it just becomes embedded in the brain, so a woman rarely gives the message(s) a second or conscious thought. She just seems to act on the message automatically as if it were true! For instance, you automatically understand what is meant by "being a good girl" or "boys don't cry." Once absorbed, these messages act as subtle ongoing influences on girls and women. Double bind messages help explain the emotional climate in which girls are raised and in which women currently live.

In her book *Beyond the Double Bind: Women and Leadership*, Kathleen Jamieson notes that a double bind offers two and only two alternatives, with one or both of these alternatives punishing the person being offered them. In her view, a double bind is a strategy always used by those with power against those without, with women, as a group, usually the individuals without the power. Double binds draw their power from their capacity to simplify the complex ways people relate; they are problematic especially when the only options are irreconcilable opposites.[4]

Consider this example. A woman is taught to project an image to men that is "soft" and feminine enough that she won't be called a lesbian, but the same image can't be so feminine that she won't be taken seriously by men. Most women live by such "rules" as if these rules are reality; unfortunately, many women do not recognize that these rules represent only one way of thinking. Instead women just get used to believing that these rules are reality, or just "the way the world is."[5]

A woman is caught in such a tangle of mixed messages she may feel unable to "do the right thing." How can she possibly respond to both messages simultaneously and experience self-confidence and a sense of competence? Obviously, she cannot. Double binds insidiously erode self-confidence. What results is a loss of personal power and diminished sense of self that results in self-hatred . . . self-hatred is the basis of hurtful behavior. Consequently double binds act as hidden yet strong influences that contribute to women hurting other women.

It is particularly difficult to live from a place of choice if a woman is not consciously aware of what she believes and how she responds to peer or societal messages. And if she can't fight the messages and the binds in which she is entrapped, then she is likely to try and break free of the binds in some other way. Women's efforts to break these binds often result in hostility and hurtful behavior toward other women.

Double binds cut across culture, ethnicity, and diversity. Women of color experience even more complexly layered and interwoven double binds; however, an in-depth exploration of binds intersecting with culture, ethnicity, and diversity is beyond the scope of our book.

Call it what you will—double bind, *Catch-22*, a "no-win" situation, the "no-choice" choice—these phrases all describe a situation that presents two equally undesirable alternatives. To expose the emotional climate in which a female child is born, a girl is raised, and a woman lives her life, we highlight several common double binds experienced by women in United States culture.

The Original Sin of Being Female

Anne Wilson Schaef, in her book *Women's Reality*, described *"the original sin of being female,"* and it is the first, most basic, and the most insidious of the double binds. This hidden bind is the least conscious to women. Shaef coined *"the original sin of being female"* to describe how females are not only deeply conditioned to feel inferior to men, but also to feel as if being born female is "bad." *Just by being born female a girl is seen as inferior, damaged, and that there is something innately wrong with her.*[6] This idea can become seamlessly ingrained into a girl's personal belief system early within her family life.

Before my (Erika's) birth, my parents opted out of knowing whether they were having a girl or boy. Yet throughout my mother's pregnancy with me I was told that my father continuously talked about how I would be born a male, and there was tremendous pressure on my mother to produce a son. Upon seeing I was a girl, a few minutes after my arrival my maternal grandmother said to my mother, "Don't worry…the next one will be a boy!" Eighteen months later my brother was born and my father joyously stated to my mother, "I am going to buy you the biggest diamond ring!" She had produced a son and the birth, in particular of a baby boy, called for a celebration. These stories were replayed with constancy throughout my youth and their stinging words never left me. Though the stories were told over laughter, the laughter never took away the feeling of being devalued. I had always been aware of feeling "less than" my brother because he was born male and I was born female. Over the years, I internalized the messages associated with being a girl and now, much later, I can see how I diminished and undervalued my own sense of competence as a result.

Kathleen Jamieson calls this bind the **bind of equality or difference**. Those in power (men) are identified as the winners and those who lack the power (women) are the losers. A woman is seen as a defective version of a man, and, as a consequence, there is no way to be viewed as competent. Women are considered subordinate whether they claim to be different from men or the same as them.[7] Listen to the conversation I (Erika) overheard recently at a local coffee shop and how easily and early in life these messages are learned.

A mother was buying coffee for herself and milk for her two young children. Her daughter appeared to be around five years old and her son about six. Neither of her children was enthusiastic about drinking milk; the mother tolerated her daughter's refusal to drink it, yet she continued to insist that her son drink the milk by repeatedly saying, "You need to drink your milk so that you can grow up and be strong, just like Popeye." When the boy used the argument that his sister was not drinking her milk, his mother stated, "But Susie is a girl and only boys need to grow up and be strong." Then I (Erika) watched the little boy gulp down his milk with great enthusiasm.

Anne Schaef suggests that when women say to each other that they do not like or trust each other, what they are really saying is that we do not like ourselves, and this comment can be expanded to "I do not like femaleness."[8] Hurtful behavior between women is easily observed and condoned in United States culture. If you are uncertain about this, just take a look at the latest "catfight" magazine headlines, commercials, or television promos and see how they use hostility between women to sell their product, service, or show. Hurtful behavior is often more readily apparent than close, loving bonds.

Schaef initially suggested that the dislike and mistrust among women originates with the original sin (born female and innately inferior to men), and because a woman's identity is dependent on validation by men and not women, women attacking each other becomes commonplace. Often when a girl or woman sees another woman seeking or getting a lot of attention from a man, she discredits or devalues her in some way.

Any attempt a woman makes to shed herself from feeling inferior seems to require some kind of validation and acknowledgement from men that she is special and/or different from other women. When a woman is validated by men, she feels like her self-worth has been enhanced, and she can consider herself different from other women; women who are not validated in the same manner can then be classified as being innately inferior to her.[9]

Most women describe having close and loving relationships with female friends, relatives, or co-workers, yet some argue that women often do not like or trust one another. Despite advances for women's rights made much earlier by the women's movement and general acceptance in society, dislike and distrust of other women, at times subtle and at other times blatant, has unquestionably remained. Ever notice how quickly women "trash-talk" another woman once she has left the room? Women seem to feel relatively safe attacking other women, sometimes even women considered close friends.

As we listened to women's stories, many women told us they would rather have male friends than female friends because they found it easier to relate to men. They said their female friends were "too catty" or competitive, they didn't trust them, and it "just hurt too much" to be friends with women.

We had a recent conversation with Carrie, a professional make-up artist, who works in an upscale department store where women routinely schedule appointments to have their makeup professionally applied. While discussing our book, Carrie told us how frequently women refuse to have their hair and makeup done by a woman and instead insist on having it done by a man. Women making this request were quite vocal about their beliefs and fears that if a woman was doing the work as opposed to a man, the female professional would intentionally make them look less attractive.

Let's go back to the earlier example with Emma. She was upset because she found her boyfriend Mark flirting with Heather. Emma reacted by attempting to defame Heather's reputation rather than by talking about her angry feelings directly with Mark. Because Emma placed Mark on a pedestal, it was easier to attack Heather than risk the loss of Mark's attention. Teenage girls attending Erika's workshops described themselves as very vocal and expressive, yet they also described feeling they had no right to stand up to male friends or boyfriends. These girls have already absorbed the idea that their worth is not equal to boys. They found it much easier and safer to attack their girlfriends.

The original sin of being born female (*by being born female, girls and women are seen as inferior, damaged, subordinate, or that something is innately wrong with them*) is the foundational bind on which all other binds follow. Because the experience of inferiority starts at birth, on its own this bind sets girls and women up for failure.

The bind appears innately unsolvable and is the beginning of the self-hatred witnessed in girls and women. How can it be possible for a girl or woman to develop high self-esteem and a good sense of herself as she matures? How can she possibly achieve or reach her fullest potential and feel good about it along the way? Because this bind starts at birth, it sets the tone for how most girls are socialized, and it marks the beginning of the path, one often filled with self-hatred, that a girl follows as she develops into a woman who oppresses other women.

The Double Bind of Emotional Expression

Women live in a culture that continuously sends out contradictory messages. Many women believe that if they perform really well (e.g. like getting good grades or being thorough and efficient at work) and are seen as too smart, they are criticized; if they perform poorly and are not smart enough, they are shamed. Hidden pressures against being authentic emerge out of contradictory messages that exist about weight, beauty, intelligence, assertiveness, and a whole range of other attributes and qualities. If a female is beautiful she is seen as a threat by other females, which is a negative . . . but if she isn't attractive she can be seen as defective or unfeminine, also a negative experience. Parents, peers, and all forms of media perpetuate contradictory messages that have negative, adverse effects that leave girls and women feeling isolated, depressed, and lonely.

The first double bind, the sin of being born female, is the most serious bind a woman experiences. It is closely linked to the experience of self-hatred (as subtle or blatant as it may be) and to hurting other women. Women experience several other binds; they include ones that relate to emotional expression, assertiveness, shame or silence, beauty, and views of what it means to be a healthy adult.

How women or men express emotion in a given situation often is affected by how they are expected to behave in that situation. Society has endorsed certain characteristics as healthy and it has established certain rules regarding how, when, and by whom particular emotions should and should not be expressed. Even young children are aware that there are rules when it comes to displaying certain types of emotions. D. W. Birnbaum and colleagues found that preschool children associate emotions such as happiness, sadness, and fear with women and they associate the emotion of anger with men. Adult men and women likewise associate happiness and fear with girls and women, and anger with boys and men. Generally speaking, it is much more acceptable to observe women outwardly express feelings of happiness and sadness and men to outwardly express feelings of anger.[10, 11]

The **double bind of emotional expression** means that both emotional expressiveness and emotional control are negatively evaluated. So if a woman expresses herself in a manner too different from what is socially expected, she can expect to be met with negative reactions from others.[12] In United States culture, women are stereotypically seen as "emotional," and often these emotional reactions are devalued and viewed as being "hysterical." However, when a female does not express any kind of emotion she is also devalued because she is not acting in line with the expectations of a stereotypical female. For instance, women who fail to express emotion in a given situation where that emotion is expected (e.g. being angry about being slapped in the face) or who are overly expressive of an emotion even when it is expected (e.g. directly expressing anger at a friend or colleague) are negatively evaluated. Here is what Candice said about her experience.

Candice, a woman in a workshop group, was in her mid-thirties. She is younger than her two outgoing sisters and grew up feeling extremely shy. While growing up she was constantly bullied by other girls about her shyness and awkward appearance. Candice began studying acting at age ten and found it to be a positive outlet; she felt safe acting in front of large audiences. Eventually, she grew out of her shyness and evolved into a capable and confident actress. She told us that the more successful and outspoken she became the more women became nasty and hurtful toward her. She stated that even successful women with whom she worked undermined her and were vicious in their gossip about her. Here is a clear example where Candice was teased as child for being withdrawn and shy while conversely as an adult she was put down for being confident, assertive, and successful.

Similar to what many other women have experienced, I (Erika) was caught in this double bind. As I matured, I was told to behave like a "little lady", guidance that included being quiet, showing no anger and deference to others. There were times when I was admonished for this type of behavior and told that I "was such a girl" and that I needed to "stop crying all the time." Alternatively, when I asserted myself and acted similar to what was deemed appropriate behavior for a male, I was told that "children should be seen and not heard" and to "calm down."

The double bind of emotional expression locks girls and women into inescapable "no-win" situations and these unspoken social rules can prevent women from being genuine and authentic with others.

Something to Think About

Think of times you held yourself back from expressing your genuine feelings based on fears of how you would be perceived or treated.

In what situations did it feel *safe* to respond the way you wanted?

In what situations did it feel *unsafe* to respond the way you wanted?

How much does your fear guide your response to various life situations?

To what degree are you compromising how you want to express yourself in the world?

Double Bind of Silence vs. Shame

Anastasia, a woman in our group, stated that when she would talk about work frustrations or about some of the issues she was experiencing with her supervisor, she was viewed as "rocking the boat." However, when she encountered a situation in which she did not express her concerns for fear of being dubbed a complainer, she felt as though she was powerless and had no control in the situation. Anastasia felt caught. She did not know where to turn or how to make the situation better, and it affected her relationships and feelings about her work experience.

Closely related to the double bind of emotional expression is a double bind that Kathleen Jamieson describes as the ***bind of silence or shame***. She suggests that silence is an outward sign of submission to persons in authority, so that if a woman remains silent or speaks submissively, then women are able to "purchase protection."[13]

What does purchase protection mean? If a woman remains silent, she is (allegedly) being protected from attack, humiliation, rejection, shaming, or exclusion by others, whether they are men or women. However, the more she remains silent, the more she fits the stereotypical view of a passive, subordinate woman; consequently, she risks being ignored and dismissed.[14] Often when women speak out they are frequently considered bossy or are called nags, shrews, or bitches, anything to question the value of their remarks. The intended effect is one of quieting, shutting down, or silencing women.

Both men and women engage in such name-calling and personality attacks. What many women don't realize is that anytime an expressive woman is condemned, no matter who does the condemning, then other women experience both obvious and hidden pressures to remain silent with her.

Something to Think About

How have you been treated by others when you have voiced your views?

Did others support you or were there efforts designed to silence you?

Were these efforts to silence you obvious to you and others or were they covert?

Have you kept yourself from speaking out based on concerns you would be shamed, humiliated, or excluded?

In what types of situations or settings does it feel comfortable to express your perspective?

In what types of situations or settings do you keep your views to yourself?

What effect did these responses have on your willingness to freely express your views or your concerns?

What do you do now?

A woman may be unaware these double bind pressures are actually influencing her, though all of these elements contribute either subtly or directly to her experience of self-confidence and competence. Absent awareness of the binds influencing her life, and having no where to turn to make sense of these messages or cast them aside, she either turns against herself or against one who is most like her . . . another woman.

Something to Think About

> Think of the hidden and obvious influence double binds have on your self-confidence, sense of competence, and how you express yourself in the world. Notice their effect on you. They act like invisible forces creating emotional pressure within. Unless you are aware of the pressure and think consciously about how you want to relate with other women, the emotional pressure can result in hurtful behavior toward women, especially because it is much harder to address and challenge the real culprits—continuing sexist attitudes and behavior or negative media influences. And it is harder still if you try to counter these forces alone.

Double Bind of Competence and Assertiveness

Double binds cut across how women express themselves in conversation and they also influence women's actions or behavior, including personal and professional choices and risks women take. Many working women who attended our trainings claimed that while at their respective places of employment they were sanctioned on their jobs if they acted either too "womanly" or too "manly." If they behaved in any way that appeared masculine-like, they were considered unfeminine. If they acted more feminine, they were considered ineffective or too passive, and then whatever they had to contribute wasn't taken seriously. Many agreed that when men are assertive they enjoy a reputation of being "go-getters," while assertive women are instead considered "domineering," "ball-busting," or "bitchy." They described feeling that if they behaved passively or dependent, they would be devalued and rejected by others.

Kathleen Jamieson described two inextricably linked double binds that help explain the plight of the women above. The first bind suggests that *women who are considered feminine will be judged incompetent, and women who are considered competent will be judged as unfeminine.* The effect of this bind is further intensified when people level "charges" that powerful women must be closeted lesbians, which of course denigrates women even further.[15] Power over others only works when the persons in power describe those who behave outside the norm as deviant or lesser than.

Consider that two of the most powerful women in the United States, Hillary Clinton and Oprah Winfrey, have both experienced repeated attacks alleging that they are lesbian. These accusations continue despite a respective long-term marriage and a relationship.

⚭

Bind of Womb or Brain

The related bind is the *bind of the womb or brain.* Over time women have been identified as bodies (or wombs) as opposed to minds and brains. This bind suggests women can exercise either their bodies or brains, but not both, and clearly not both simultaneously![16]

Throughout history women who chose not to have children were considered defective and seen typically by society as either an asexual spinster or a lesbian; a married woman who chose not to have children and worked instead was presumed to be self-centered and aggressive and that she purposely sacrificed her mothering role for her profession.[17]

Men have been stereotyped as "thinkers" whereas women are known for their feelings. In fact, women are treated as if their bodies are in charge and men are treated as if they are ruled by their "logical" thinking minds. Think about how many women were kept out of responsible positions (including political office) for years because of concerns tied to menstrual cycles and emotional instability. It's easy to see how assumptions that educating a woman's brain/mind would make her less desirable to men. This bind continues to have much traction.

In a radio interview with Carla J. Christofferson, the co-owner of the Los Angeles Sparks (the women's professional basketball team) and managing partner of a large Los Angeles law firm, Carla described how many female lawyers were unfortunately "dumbing themselves down" with men they were dating. The women would initially tell the men that they were working at the law firm but would not specify the role (as in lawyer), instead preferring to have their dates think they were working at the firm in administrative roles. In many cases, the women were also more financially successful than the men.

On a day-to-day basis women may be less aware of the negative influence of double binds. Consider just how engrained these biases are and how effectively these double binds operate, as described in the research study below. The strength of these views can still be seen.

Researchers believe that both men and women are socialized to believe women are less intelligent than men. In the classic study *"Are Women Prejudiced against Women?"* researcher Philip A. Goldberg asked men and women to evaluate the intelligence, persuasiveness, and style of a set of identical essays, written either by John or Joan. With the exception of the name and proper pronoun, Joan's essays received consistently lower ratings from both men and women than John's.[18] Goldberg's original findings have been confirmed by other studies.[19, 20] The resulting tragedy is that a female begins to believe and then acts and behaves in accordance with these stereotypes, generally remaining unaware of the beliefs binding her.

Something to Think About

Have you ever "dumbed yourself down"?

Have you ever "dumbed yourself down" or made yourself appear less attractive because you didn't want your girlfriends to see you as too threatening?

Do you "dumb yourself down" around female co-workers/ colleagues or around your women friends?

What effect does "dumbing down" have on how you relate with or treat other women?

Do you still "dumb yourself down"? If so, why are you making this choice?

How many of you have been told to let a boy or man win when you have been competing against him in a competitive task or game?

Have you deferred, letting the boy or man win, even though you could have won?

Have you ever been told not to be more intelligent than the boys or men around you?

What effect does "dumbing down" and "sexing up" for boys and men have on your self-esteem?

"Looking-Glass Self" Double Bind

Charles Horton Cooley first described the idea of *The Looking-Glass Self.*[21] According to this idea, a woman views herself through others' perceptions to help establish her own sense of identity. Researchers King-to Yeung and John Levi Martin described three main components of the Looking-Glass Self.[22] They suggested that a woman imagines how she appears to others, then imagines the judgment of that appearance, and, finally, she develops her self through the judgments of others. Thus, a woman is strongly influenced by those with whom she associates and also by those she deems important.

I (Joan) teach in masters and doctoral graduate psychology programs and have contact with many women in their mid-twenties. I am aware that several of these women put themselves in financial debt and at financial risk simply to feel similar to the persons they admire. The women in their mid-twenties, in turn, treat other women poorly and exclude them when they don't live up to the same styles or behaviors they themselves have been emulating.

A mother of a thirteen-year-old girl from a "Mean Girls . . . Meaner Women" workshop that I (Erika) recently presented told us that her daughter Jasmine was having a difficult time because Jasmine was constantly judging herself based on how she thought her friends viewed her. Jasmine believed that her friends thought she was unattractive and didn't know how to dress well or trendy enough, and as a result she was constantly putting herself down. She used the continued negative judgments by her "friends" as fodder for her own personal attacks against herself. Jasmine was struggling to fit into her peer group. Jasmine's mother relayed how frustrating this experience was for her as well. As Jasmine's mother, she felt powerless to impact the intense social pressure on Jasmine to look and act a certain way.

Despite Cooley's impressions in the early 1900s, his idea remains applicable to girls and women today. A woman uses friendships and other social relationships to help define her sense of self.

While everyone relies on some feedback from others about themselves, the bind associated with the *looking-glass self* is when a girl or woman *overly relies* on others to define her own sense of self—something we witness in girls' and women's behavior as they try to follow in the exact footsteps of their chosen idols. In the extreme, a woman may dismiss her own knowledge and wisdom about what is best for her, sometimes putting her own health or welfare at risk. If she is absent a strong sense of self, she may lash out at others for having what she desires for herself, hating in others what she hates in herself, or attacking women she perceives less well off than herself.

Something to Think About

How do you rely on the views of others to help you decide what you like and dislike?

How do you rely on the views of others to decide who you should be friends with?

How do you rely on the views of others to help define your sense of identity?

Do other's perceptions of you influence your attitudes, beliefs, or actions?

What do you do when the pressure is great to behave a certain way even though it doesn't fit your own belief system or values?

Does this pressure ever turn into attacks upon yourself? If so, what do you say to yourself?

Does this pressure ever turn into anger and attacks on others (including others who are making choices different from you or your friends?

Beauty and the Bind

Dr. Deborah Cox and her colleagues have been studying United States "beauty culture" in order to understand how beauty is experienced by women and between women, including how it is experienced across several aspects of diversity that involve African-American, Hispanic, disabled, aging, lesbian, and beauty extremes (pretty and un-pretty) women. She describes the *beauty double bind*.[23]

> We're calling this a double bind because in the Beauty Culture dance, women cannot admit trying to look a particular way or caring very much about appearance or body. If they admit caring or concern, they risk their status in the competitive dance; part of the competition is a race toward appearing the most noncompetitive and the most unconcerned about beauty. When women master the art of appearing unconcerned while having high levels of physical beauty and thinness, they win.

She continues by noting:

> This competition and dance are stealthy, covert operations. Women can in some ways go undetected, yet other women seem to know (intuitively) what is going on. Most have a hard time defining it. Some admit they feel it. Others deny and minimize their experience. Appearing not to care about sparring between women seems to also add points to a woman's status. At the same time, this is a double bind because not talking makes the distance greater between the women. So while women may take themselves "out of relationship" [by not talking with other women about this issue] in order to protect their standing with other women, or perhaps with men, they do so at their own loss of connection with support, information, and nurturance from other women. The competition also incorporates elements beyond beauty including: career status, wealth, prestige,

relationship success, children and family, etc. Many women in our study talked about feeling isolated from other women, along with not having woman friends and not being able to trust women.[24]

Our culture teaches girls and women not to be competitive with each other. What Dr. Cox is saying about the *beauty culture* bind is that girls and women often feel very competitive with each other over such issues as attractiveness, thinness, intelligence, and quality boyfriends or male partners. Women are taught to be humble and not proud. Women, in fact, are highly competitive with each other, yet they simultaneously deny that this competition has any importance to them.

Dr. Cox related a story from one of her groups where a woman actively denied feeling competitive with other women around issues of beauty. A few days after the group met, one young woman called Dr. Cox to tell her that she had been dishonest during the group meeting. She tearfully described that she felt enormous pressure to be competitive with women. She stated that she struggled with her weight and acted like she could eat anything she wanted to and not gain weight. She was ashamed to tell the truth in front of her friends.[25] Women are especially fearful of talking honestly about the competition involved with beauty and attractiveness.

This topic is complex. From very young ages girls are taught to wear makeup, dress in provocative ways, and do most anything that will accentuate female sexuality and attractiveness; regardless of age, females are encouraged to use sexuality to gain access to resources (men, status, power). Clearly opportunities for closeness with other women are lost because women are afraid to be authentic with each other.

Paradox of the Healthy Adult

The landmark study conducted by I. Broverman and her colleagues in 1970 is widely recognized as one of the most influential and important studies on sex bias and the judgment of mental health. In the study, male and female psychologists, psychiatrists, and social workers were asked to identify characteristics of healthy men, healthy women, and healthy adults (no sex specified). Overall, participants described *healthy men and healthy adults as having the same qualities,* yet they described healthy women as having very different qualities than healthy adults.[26] A double standard of mental health existed for women; *for a woman to be seen as mentally healthy she must be feminine, yet not like an adult and not like a man.*

Healthy women were portrayed as more submissive, less competitive, less independent, and more emotional, while *healthy adults* were active, independent, and logical. It was actually *impossible to be seen as both a healthy adult and a healthy woman.* Study participants were significantly less likely to attribute traits that characterize healthy adults to a woman; instead they were likely to attribute these traits to a man.

Serious implications can be drawn from the stereotyping described in this study; to be considered an *unhealthy adult,* women must act as women are "supposed" to act (e.g. conform to the female sex role stereotype); to be considered an *unhealthy woman,* women must act as men are supposed to act—which is even more confusing because men are seen as healthy when they act the exact same way! We call this double bind *the paradox of the healthy adult*.

The researchers posited that there are different standards of mental health for women and men, including tacit and hidden assumptions that dependency and passivity are normal for women. The researchers concentrated on the complex challenges that women face appearing feminine while functioning as healthy adults in an adult world. They found it was more socially desirable to have masculine traits, except, of course, if a woman started to appear too masculine.[27] Pretty confusing, and perhaps a bit hard to digest.

Many of the original views of a healthy male and healthy adult have held over time. More recently, researchers Susan R. Seem and M. Diane Clark found that the traditional masculine and feminine gender role stereotypes remain largely unchanged, with the exception that now a healthy adult woman possesses both nurturing and competency traits.[28]

Seem and Clark noted views of a healthy adult woman differed significantly from those of a healthy adult man and a healthy adult. Yet again, a healthy adult man was viewed as similar to a healthy adult. [29] They suggest there may be two different standards of mental health, one for healthy women and one for healthy men.[30] However, the two standards have remained highly traditional in terms of gender role stereotypes.

What does this later research mean? To be a mentally healthy adult, a woman must exhibit traditionally feminine characteristics. She cannot be like a man, nor can she exhibit masculine characteristics. However, the conception of today's woman includes competency characteristics of a man—so she should both be like him (in only very small ways) and not be like him simultaneously to be a healthy adult![31]

For a woman to be considered healthy she must adjust to and accept the social norms for women, even though these behaviors are considered less healthy. Thus, she is placed in an inconceivable bind . . . forced to choose between displaying "positive" characteristics considered desirable for men and adults, yet simultaneously at risk of compromising her "femininity." Or she has the option to behave like a stereotypical woman and accept her (generally) devalued, passive, lower-class status. The consequences of behaving like a "healthy male", meaning acting ambitious, adventurous, assertive, and competitive, are that women can be accused of being non- feminine and acting just like a man. Effectiveness and manliness are seen as synonyms.[32] Women who live outside the norm of feminine stereotypes or who exhibit personal qualities of being active, independent, and logical may experience a backlash by other women. Unfortunately, these binds leave very little room for a woman to live authentically and express her genuine thoughts and feelings.

Double Binds in Real Life

Double Binds and Lesbian Women

From work on "tomboyism," Lee Zevy, author of *Sissies and Tomboys: Gender Nonconformity and Homosexual Childhood,* noted that lesbian women experience double binds. She describes tomboyism as a fluid emotional experience sandwiched between male and female social norms. Though this period in a young girl's life is often considered insignificant, it is a time when girls can learn nurturing and social skills, skills that can facilitate acceptance into a female world; simultaneously girls can engage in activities that involve adventure, fighting, competition, and risk-taking, all behaviors that can help them achieve self-confidence, self-esteem, and personal power in adulthood.[33]

However, a woman who exhibits qualities or traits attributed to masculinity is considered unhealthy, damaged, and even more inferior than a heterosexual woman who behaves in a stereotypical manner (e.g. passive, quiet, deferential to men). Interesting to note that the best way to insult a man is to associate him to girls or women or to attribute feminine characteristics to him; the best way to insult a woman is suggest she is more like a man.

A lesbian woman is likely to have an even greater experience of being an "outsider", functioning competently alongside men in their previously established domains (e.g. male dominated professions) yet still bound by rigidly defined female gender roles and behaviors. Several double binds are at work here, including binds of expression, shame vs. silence, competence and assertiveness, and the paradox of the healthy adult.

Double Binds and Play

The *original sin of being female* and *looking-glass self* double binds help decipher young girls' behaviors. Young girls see themselves in the toys with which they play. In May 2007, a new doll was marketed hyping the to-be-released *Spider Man III* film.[34] The "Mary Jane Comiquette" was unveiled (literally and figuratively speaking) to the public, sporting generous cleavage, tight, low-cut jeans, and a very exposed pink thong peeking out from inside her jeans. If this image isn't disturbing enough, the advertisement for the doll depicted Mary Jane bending over a tub scrubbing "Spidey's" iconic superhero gear. This doll delivered a false, yet potent message that females should be both sexual beings for the gratification of others as well as subservient (a maid/slave). With this doll, a young girl is exposed to the bind of being a caretaker for others and a sexual object, absent links to her intelligence and sense of identity. Girls are bombarded with messages effective at maintaining stereotypes of inferiority, heightened sexuality, absence of critical thought, and servitude to men.

Following the release of the film *The Fantastic Four*, Mattel marketed "The Invisible Woman Barbie" doll.[35] The Invisible Woman Barbie was the film character who was accidentally exposed to radiated cosmic rays during a rocket test flight. The three other characters are male and have superpowers that range from Mr. Fantastic, who can stretch his body, to Pilot Ben Grimm, who can turn himself into a super-strong rock creature. The Invisible Woman is able to render herself or other people or objects invisible. Take serious note, there is a double bind message embedded here. While the

Invisible Woman Barbie is beautiful, with blonde hair and sporting a skin-tight blue suit, her "superpower" is that she is invisible (and in the case of the doll, her arms are invisible). Quite an interesting double bind message: she has a superpower . . . it's just that she and it (the superpower) are invisible. Not only does this doll serve as a "looking-glass self" reference point, it also delivers the message that girls should be beautiful, yet simultaneously maintain their invisibility. It provides an example of the *original sin of being female* operating quietly (and perhaps invisibly) at work.

Amanda, a nineteen-year-old woman in one of the workshops, was tall, thin, and had long, bleached blonde hair. She was going to college part-time and was struggling to be a successful actress/model, as are many other women in Los Angeles. She told us that when she was growing up she asked her mom for a new Barbie doll every birthday and Christmas. She said that she had over a hundred Barbies and their respective accessories by the time she was twelve. Amanda talked about her desire to grow up and "be" Barbie . . . to look, talk, and dress like her. By the time she was sixteen Amanda had dyed her dark brown hair bleach blonde and subsequently developed an eating disorder in order to be thin like her Barbie dolls. Amanda was quite tearful as she talked about the pressures she felt to act like the people she saw in the news. She said she continues to feel ongoing pressure to be like them, especially given the images and messages she is confronted with on a daily basis.

Girls learn about sharing and communication as they play with dolls, yet many of today's dolls seem to play up negative and conflicting stereotypes. While many girls grew up emulating Barbie, girls, including pre-schoolers, now play with the hugely popular and highly sexualized Bratz or Hannah Montana dolls. In 2004, the BBC news announced that the Bratz doll oversold Barbie and become the number one doll in the United Kingdom.

The appeal for Bratz over Barbie relates to their unique looks . . . thick lips and diverse skin tones, a step forward given our multiethnic population. However, the hyper-sexualized dolls are featured dressed in revealing outfits and engaging in sexually risky behaviors. The Bratz Secret Date collection featured the doll sneaking out of the house to go meet a mysterious boy she did not know. The Twiinz dolls, Phoebe and Roxxi, released in 2004, features twin Bratz dolls; however, one is dressed more angel-like while the other looks more devilish. Consider the message: a girl must be angel-like in public while devilish privately in the bedroom. Other collections include Bikini Bratz, Strut It, Wild Life Safari, and Nighty Nite.

This collection of dolls once again sends an array of confusing messages. Girls can be different (which is empowering) yet they still have to use their sexuality to succeed . . . again a no-win situation! Or the message is that girls should look like the dolls . . . yet don't be too pretty or other girls may become jealous and see you as competition.

Double Binds and TV Programming

The E! television reality series *The Girls Next Door* premiered in August 2005 and focused on Hugh Hefner and three young girlfriends who lived with him at the Playboy Mansion.[36] The series was immediately a ratings hit. Surprisingly, their number one viewer is not boys or men, but young women (*Larry King Live* interview on May 18, 2007). Perhaps viewers believe they too can use their sexuality to gain money, fame, and fortune (via a man) and they see the "girls next door" as role models. Women in this program, literally, serve at the pleasure of men. This show offers just one example of a program where double bind messages can be observed. With *The Girls Next Door* series, you can see the womb vs. brain double bind operating; in this case, women as wombs take center stage. Some telling episode titles for *The Girls Next Door* include: "Under the Covers" and "Clue-less" (Season One); "Mutiny on the Booty," "Sleepwear Optional," and "Heavy Petting" (Season Two); "My Bare Lady" and "Dangerous Curves" (Season Three); and "Unveilings" (Season Four).

A Last Look at Double Binds

As most young girls develop their sense of self and identity, they experience countless social pressures to behave in a traditional or stereotypically feminine manner; girls simultaneously experience other pressures in the form of societal double binds. These double binds are multiply layered and inextricably linked together. Anne Schaef's conception of "*the original sin*" for females, that an individual born female is innately inferior based on being female, puts girls and women at an immediate disadvantage; being female necessarily dictates an experience of inferiority.[37] Not only does being female determine inferior status, as a woman reaches adulthood, it means she is perceived as an "*unhealthy adult.*"

As girls mature they face double binds that involve expression, assertiveness, competence, and visibility. If a female is assertive and speaks her mind, she can be seen as acting more like a male; if she says nothing or is passive (under-expressive) she is seen as stereotypically female. Since most girls grow up experiencing double bind messages about how they should communicate, they often do not learn how to properly express their emotion.

It is often unhealthy for a woman in this culture to allow herself to be seen as expressive, independent, and logical, and a woman who possesses these qualities may experience a backlash by other women. Thus, expression, behavior, and visibility each involve a woman facing and struggling with choices about her degree of assertiveness. Speaking and behaving passively tie her into a stereotypically feminine role beset by more dismissal and invisibility. Speaking and behaving assertively means she could be considered "too" visible, and then she confronts being defined as too manly. Assertiveness and competence aren't seen as genuine options as these actions can lead to experiences of shame or exclusion instead.

It can be difficult for women to be their authentic selves, filled with high self-esteem and a sense that they can do anything they set out to accomplish. Instead they are in the unfortunate position of being reinforced "for acting in the very ways that objectify" and constrict them and ultimately "render them less significant, less visible, and less in control".[38] Given this complex set of mixed messages, entrapping a woman at every turn, with no fair and safe outlet for her anger and frustration, just what is a woman to do?

Women turn this anger and aggression inward first, living either with a low level of self-hatred (like a mild, lingering depression) or self-hatred that manifests in a self-destructive manner (e.g. eating disorders, drug abuse, or self-mutilating behavior) until it eventually moves outward toward others. Regardless of the form it takes, these insidious double binds act as both a precursor and contributor to self-hatred; self-hatred is a key link to a girl's aggression toward other girls and a woman's hurtful behavior toward other women. A woman often finds it difficult to challenge the specific beliefs or source of these messages; instead she more commonly attacks someone like herself . . . another woman.

Something to Think About

Double bind messages have influenced you even if you have not been aware of their impact. They limit your choices and may affect your honesty with yourself and authenticity with others. Understand how you are influenced by them, how to critically analyze what they convey, and how these demands may act as pressure for women to be hurtful to other women so you can be more aware of the challenges you face being just who you want to be in this world.

Your Experience with Double Bind Messages

- While growing up you hate wearing dresses or skirts and love to play sports but others tell you that you behave too masculine.

- While growing up you love playing with dolls and generally behave passive and shy; others tell you that you need to be stronger and more assertive and that you behave too feminine.

- You excel in school, sports, your career, and other areas and your female friends begin to turn on you and tell you that you are "too perfect."

- You must be attractive but not overly attractive, as other females might feel threatened by your attractiveness.

- You must be sexually appealing, sensual, and alluring, but if you are too sexual or sexually active with males and/or females you may be deemed a slut or whore.

- You are seen as critical, domineering, or aggressive when you speak out about some issue or concern.

- You don't speak out about a situation or issue you feel is wrong for fear of being called pushy or dominating; instead you are called passive, apathetic, or docile.

- In your employment setting you stand up for what you feel is right and put your needs first yet others call you either a "bitch" or a "ball-buster."

- You are a working mother and others call you selfish for choosing work over your child.

- You are a full-time stay-at-home mom and others call you lazy for not working.

- You decide to put your needs first and take care of yourself, and others deem you "too confident" or "selfish."

- What other double bind messages have you experienced?

Chapter VI

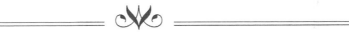

Belonging to the Girls Club:
What It Really Means

Double binds act as hidden forces that may compel a woman to make certain choices about how to live her life. Yet decisions, especially early in life, are often made without full knowledge of what elements are influencing them. Double bind messages are experienced very early (around ages two and three) and exert subtle influences; consequently, these messages can be hard to decipher or challenge. Girls and women experience messages about *gender* in a manner similar to double binds. Both types of messages exert pressure and may influence women to behave in hurtful ways toward each other.

Sex or Gender?

Sex and *gender* are often used interchangeably. *Sex,* in the field of psychology, refers to the aspects that define a person as a biological female or biological male and is determined by genetic make-up, internal reproductive organs, the organizational structure of the brain, and external genitalia. *Gender* involves assumed roles (e.g. stay-at-home mom, career woman, engineer, athlete, leader, administrator) and personality characteristics (shy, assertive, demure, risk-taker, aggressive). Children learn about gender from societal and cultural messages about how one should act or function in the world. These messages exert tremendous influence on females, and these influences are considered just as important as a person's biological and genetic makeup. Gender has also been described as the psychological experience of one's biological sex.

Absorbing and Internalizing Culture: Developing a Gender Identity

Gender identity evolves out of a girl's ability to recognize her sex difference from boys (e.g. I am a girl); it emerges early in life. A girl has the ability to understand differences between gender-linked physical traits such as faces at around one year of age. A growing sense of gender identity emerges around two years of age when she begins to use gender (girl, boy) to label other people, and it is typically one of the very first descriptors she uses to identify herself.

A girl begins to clearly acknowledge her own gender at approximately three years of age and between three and six years the gender of others is easily accomplished. Also by the age of three children are sorting through many types of differences (e.g. skin color), of which gender is only one. Before children formally enter school (again ages three and four) they are able to discern power differences between boys and girls, including how to resolve conflicts with boys differently than how they resolve them with girls.[1] At these ages children are able to understand the categories of male and female and they can differentiate both the blatant (e.g. girls shouldn't be angry) and subtle messages (disapproving looks or tone of voice) about what is considered proper or improper behavior for males and females.

Around six years of age a girl tends to form stereotypes, especially regarding social roles. She also becomes aware of cultural messages and norms regarding what it means to behave as a girl. Likewise, she learns about positive and negative stereotypes of her own sex and about boys. Beliefs adopted in early childhood form the basis of the gender roles a woman later adopts in adulthood.[2]

Something to Think About

Consider aspects typically associated to boys/men and girls/women as they cut across: *color* (bright for boys, soft muted pastel for girls); *decorating themes* (sports and action for boys, doll or fantasy for girls); *toys; clothes; types of activities* (football not for girls, dressing up not for boys); *careers; sports played; hair style and manner of dress; use of language* (e.g. swearing); and *acceptable sexual behavior or activity* and *human bodily functions.*[3]

From birth and infancy through adulthood girls are generally socialized into obeying traditional gender roles and behaving in conventional or stereotypically feminine ways. What is considered appropriate behavior for girls and boys is imposed on most aspects of everyday life. It happens seamlessly, without well-considered thought as to how these messages influence and affect decisions in all aspects of life. A young girl understands the world and her functioning in it defined along these gender lines. She quickly adopts these values and adjusts her behavior to fit in with cultural gender norms and expectations and uses these beliefs as a template as she matures into an adult woman.

> Imagine what could happen for you if life was not categorized based on beliefs made about sex and gender or, if we stretched it further, even about the shade of your skin.

Gender beliefs operate in a manner similar to double bind messages, imposing unseen rules and influence over female (and male) behavior. Strict gender roles prevail for everyone as a result. Hidden assumptions about sex and gender find their way into everyday conversations, activities, and social institutions such as marriage, relationships, religious observation, sports, and work; they become part of each person's own belief system.[4] They include beliefs that the psychological and sexual natures of men and women are fundamentally different from each other; that men are inherently the dominant or superior sex; and that it is generally accepted that both male-female difference and male dominance are natural.[5]

In United States culture men are perceived as inherently superior to women, and the male and his experience are used as the standard or norm against which all other experiences are judged, evaluated, or valued. As a consequence of this view, any girl or woman and her respective experience(s) are automatically deviations from the male norm and inferior by consequence.[6] Belief in a male-centered culture is pervasive. It is intertwined with the "original sin" and "paradox of a healthy adult" double binds, thus strengthening the view of women as inferior and unhealthy.

Sandra Bem, author of *The Lenses of Gender*, describes how femininity and masculinity are considered as opposite ends of a single dimension of gender (*gender polarization*), so that a person must be either feminine or masculine, but not both simultaneously. She notes that there is one and only one very rigid script for how a girl or woman should be and one and only one similarly rigid script for how a man should be. Any behavior other than stereotyped or conventional femininity or masculinity is considered abnormal, deviant, or pathological.[7]

Ellie, an eighteen-year-old high school student, attended one of our talks. Ellie attended an elite private school. She said she knew that she felt different from the other girls as early as four years old. Ellie was never interested in playing with dolls like her friends did—she was more interested in playing soccer than with tea sets. If it was up to her, she would still be running around without a shirt on, just like the boys. She explained that she was always pressured to be more traditionally feminine but that was never comfortable for her—she never felt "her true self." Throughout most of her life, including now, all the other girls in school made her an outcast because she wasn't "girl" enough for them. The girls would tease her and call her names because of the way she carried herself and the way she looked; she could care less about the latest fashion and wore her hair really short. Ellie told us that she wanted to be friends with the other girls in school, but because of their teasing and bullying she always felt like she couldn't fit in with them, and she still felt out of place. She found it hard to make friends and she spent most of her time alone.

There is almost no human experience that women have or accomplish that does not have the notion of sex or sex difference attached to it.[8] This belief guides choices that include dress, leisure activities, career opportunities or careers pursued, emotional expression, expression of sexual desire, and perhaps even excelling at activities (e.g. winning in competitions with men or not showing how smart you are because "men don't like women smarter than them"). Likewise, experiences involving independence, autonomy, physical strength, power, anger, and aggression are considered gender inappropriate for females, while feelings of vulnerability ("don't cry"), dependency or need, closeness, sadness, and same-sex affection or love is seen as gender inappropriate for males.[9] Even male connection and emotional closeness is trivialized and differentiated from being gay by using phrases like "male-bonding," "man-date," and "bromance" to describe such closeness.

Two important consequences result from categorizing women and femaleness at one extreme and men and maleness at the other extreme. First, *men and women are socialized to live by mutually exclusive scripts* (guidelines or rules) for how to behave as a male or female. Mass media outlets including print, TV, movie, and advertising primarily reinforce these established scripts. Second, *any person or behavior that deviates from these well-defined scripts is considered problematic, immoral, or unnatural.* A woman who veers from these clear and predefined notions of what it means to be female is viewed as deviant from religious, scientific, and psychiatric/psychological perspectives.[10]

This last point is a key one. **Anyone who behaves outside these scripts or rules is seen as biologically and psychologically deviant** (e.g. outspoken women, lesbians). What results is the experience of enormous and sometimes unspeakable pressure for girls and women to behave in extremely narrow and culturally scripted ways, especially if they fall outside established notions of a stereotypically feminine woman.

Something to Think About

Do you behave in ways that fall outside the cultural norm of femininity? In what ways does your "*difference*" get expressed? What have people said to you? How have you been treated because of it? Have you been kept from certain opportunities because of your difference?

Everything gets both influenced and interpreted through cultural and societal influences. As a girl absorbs and adopts these views, she constructs an identity consistent with her beliefs. Strict and very narrowly defined gender roles prevent girls and women from being authentically themselves and in turn may become another influence that leads women to attack, betray, or exclude any women who deviate from these norms.

Layla, a thirty-seven-year-old woman who was one of my (Erika's) clients, was in therapy to deal with longstanding issues involved with being overweight. She described having been heavy from her late teen years through adulthood. She was still suffering greatly from numerous incidents of name calling, physical attacks, derisive laughter, and practical jokes leveled against her by female peers, based on her size and weight. As an adult, she was slow to trust others based on fears of other attacks, yet she was able to develop some friends. However, she mostly stayed at home even when asked to join others in various activities. She still insulated herself from hurtful behavior. She was preoccupied with her appearance and she generally felt isolated from women. She described feeling so different from them that she didn't even feel "womanly." She had reached a point of deep despair and realized that the only way her life could get better was if she sought help to deal with concerns relating to her appearance and other critical life issues, make key decisions, and get on with her life in a more satisfying manner.

Something to Think About

Think about people you know or have observed who fall outside cultural norms of femininity or masculinity. How do they present themselves? What do you think about them? What do others think and say about them? How do they get treated by others? How do you treat them?

Any discussion of masculinity and femininity must be tied directly to cultural and societal expectations, rules, and roles associated with being male or female, otherwise the discussion really has no meaning. Societal pressures to fit into strict gender roles, especially when they don't fit, contribute to a growing sense of self-hatred ("there must be something wrong with me") . . . self-hatred contributes to girls becoming women who may later backstab, betray, or "trash-talk" other women. Societal messages about "proper" female behavior can lead to a girl/woman feeling "less (adequate) than" other girls/women, a situation which also lends itself to a woman experiencing self-hatred and then displacing or projecting her own feelings of worthlessness onto other females. The odd twist is that when people feel inadequate or less than, they often behave in the exact opposite manner—acting superior to others and treating others poorly. Consequently, women hurt, betray, backstab, trash-talk, or exclude other women.

Our Gendered Lives

Mandy, a nineteen-year-old college student who attended a recent talk at a Greek sorority conference, told us that all throughout junior high and high school all her friends began developing breasts except her. She was so envious of her friends' blossoming figures that she tried everything to look like them, including stuffing her bra. Feeling hopeless about any real changes she begged her parents to buy her breast augmentation surgery for her high school graduation gift and her parents ultimately acquiesced. When we asked her why she made that decision at such a young age, Mandy confessed that she wanted to have her breasts enlarged because she couldn't handle feeling so jealous of other girls' curvy figures and that she wanted to be as desirable to men as her friends were. She said her friends now tell her that they "hate her" because of her breasts and they are envious of her looks.

We recently interviewed Cora Daniels, a journalist, author, and frequent TV commentator on social issues, for our Women's Inspiration Los Angeles radio show. Her book, *GhettoNation: A Journey into the Land of Bling and Home of the Shameless*, was the interview focus.[11] During the interview she described how she went out to look for Halloween costumes for her infant daughter and came across "pimp and ho" costumes that were available in newborn sizes! She said her friend found three-foot-high "pole dancing" kits for girls that are sold in toy stores. Both are excellent examples of how gender messages are easily and seamlessly woven into our culture. These messages blindly (or perhaps blatantly) acculturate girls into definitive feminine roles, with men in positions of power and privilege. The "pimp and ho" costumes and pole dancing kit suggest particular roles for girls/women and boys/men and put boys/men in a power and privilege position, as girls are socialized, from infancy (!), to cater to what men want.

Let's look at the second example a little more in depth. The pole-dancing kit was advertised to young females in 2006. The kit includes a chrome pole extendible to eight feet six inches, a "sexy dance garter," and a DVD demonstrating suggestive dance moves. The pole-dancing kit was pulled off the toys and games section of the popular Tesco store website in the United Kingdom after consumers complained. The Tesco Direct site advertised the kit with the words, "Unleash the sex kitten inside . . . simply extend the Peekaboo pole inside the tube, slip on the sexy tunes, and away you go! Soon you'll be flaunting it to the world and earning a fortune in Peekaboo Dance Dollars."

"Toys" such as these suggest to girls that being female means you must engage in sexually provocative activities at a young age for the entertainment of males. Girls are bombarded with images of sexual behavior and learn this is what it means to be female and that if you deviate from this standard then you are most certainly not a "normal" girl.

Interestingly, girls and women are often insulted and "put down" using males as the reference group ("she's too aggressive" or "too much like a man"); the strongest, most effective, and most damning insult you can level at boys or men is to say they are being more like girls, using females as a reference group ("he's a sissy" or "girlie"). One particular example of such behavior within the past few years involves the governor of California, Arnold Schwarzenegger, who chided a particular interest group by calling them "girlie men." While he was briefly criticized for his comment, the event passed and was quickly buried under other news items.

Something to Think About

> Striking, isn't it, that the worst insult you can deliver a man is to compare him or identify him with anything female? What does that say about women? Equally as important, why does this behavior remain acceptable in our culture or that it remains absent responses that stop such behavior?

Our culture clearly has ideas about what it is to be a "real male" or "real female" despite how restrictive these gender definitions are for both women and men, and these are only a few ways our culture engages in gender polarizing social practices. "The consequences of having a social definition of sex (tied to gender) leaves female and male children with the feeling that they must 'work at' being female or male—or that it is something to accomplish and never lose, as opposed to simply being something that one *is* biologically."[12]

Consider this idea of "working at" being female (a "real woman") or male (a "real man") a little further and the damage to a sense of self that can result. Sandra Bem suggests that both women and men are left with a deep sense of insecurity that they will never live up to the culturally defined gender ideal; equally as bad, girls and women and boys and men then must respectively repress feelings (disappointment, sadness, anger, competition) or natural human instincts and needs (desire for closeness, dependency, affiliation, affection). She notes the net result of such repression is that it can cause even more internal self-conflict, leading to even more gender insecurity.[13]

So rather than a girl just being able to know she is female and think no further about it, she instead must make sure her words, actions, beliefs, behaviors, and activities are congruent with what is considered "appropriately" feminine. A girl may end up feeling inadequate and insecure about being female. This constant checking can also lead to a sense of inadequacy and insecurity about her gender, because *anything outside strictly defined gender ideals is seen as deviant or alien.* That is why, for instance, strong women are labeled lesbian, and boys who exhibit more effeminate behaviors are called "sissies" and faggots, or they are labeled as gay.[14]

Though our focus is only on women at this time, please understand that these strict demands affect men too. I (Joan) attended the first National Men's Psychotherapy Conference in Los Angeles, Calif., and heard three psychologists knowledgeable about men's issues state unequivocally in agreement that the men they see in their psychotherapy practices feel inadequate and unable to live up to the stereotype of the ideal man.[15]

Gender Police:
Enforcing Deviant Gender Behavior

No doubt you are familiar with the notion of "fashion police". You know the individuals who have taken it upon themselves to evaluate and judge what people are wearing, to ensure they are in line with the latest fashion or most up-to-date trend. And watch out if they are not; shame and humiliation can result. The infamous Red Carpet at the Oscars or the Emmy Award shows stand out as the most obvious examples of television personalities "policing" fashion and "dishing" on "who was wearing what." There is a parallel notion as it relates to gender. In this case, think of it as policing gender . . . or "gender police."

Children learn and believe early that there are gender-related characteristics, attitudes, behaviors, and occupations, and they monitor their own social behavior according to society's definitions of what is masculine and what is feminine. Parents, siblings, peers, and many other responsible adults play crucial roles in shaping a child's behaviors in ways deemed appropriate for each sex, and boys and girls are often rewarded and punished for different behaviors according to their sex.

Parents choose different clothing for their children, encourage them to play with gender-typed toys, and continue to divide household chores along gender lines. Girls are frequently praised for displaying helpful and nurturing behaviors and boys are rewarded for exhibiting autonomy and independence. Boys are still admonished for displaying more "feminine" emotions such as crying ("big boys don't cry") and girls may be criticized for engaging in "male" behaviors such as physically rough play ("can't you play more nicely?"). Children watch carefully and then imitate the behaviors of same sex adults and peers; they use these observations to shape their own behavior according to what they believe is typical for girls and boys.

I (Erika) was recently standing at a card store counter waiting to complete my purchase when I overheard a mother tell her seven- or eight-year-old son that the (rather gender neutral) stuffed animals he was looking at and wanted for himself were "too girlie." The mother continued by emphasizing the point, "You don't want it. I am not going to buy you the toy and have you playing with any 'girlie' stuffed animals. They are for girls, not boys." It was only one comment by his mother, but think of the various implications of her remark and what it says about his experience of himself.

It is well established that parents model, encourage, and guide children into different activities and behaviors based on their biological sex and the cultural proscription for "proper" feminine and masculine behavior. Naturally, as children learn to monitor their own behavior, they begin evaluating, correcting, and enforcing or "policing" the behavior of their peers in relation to culturally defined "gender appropriate" ways of behaving. Likewise they learn to reject or disavow any manner of behaving that does not match their sex or the gender appropriate way to behave. Just that quickly most children smoothly and unobtrusively begin to function in a conventionally sex-typed manner themselves.

Jill, a forty-year-old woman who attended a workshop on women oppressing women that I (Erika) presented, described her parent's rigid enforcement of a family dress code. We were talking about how children are socialized into particular gender roles and learn "gender-appropriate" behaviors. Jill's parents made her wear only skirts and dresses to a wide variety of social activities because that's what girls did and that was what was expected of her. Jill wanted to dress like her older brother, who was always comfortably dressed in pants. Jill told us that this constant bickering about how she should "dress more like a girl" resulted in numerous arguments and tears about doing something that didn't feel right to her. Natasha, another participant, told us she was kept out of grade school activities and responsibilities she wanted, such as becoming a school crossing guard, and she was kept from playing certain sports simply because she was a girl. Both Jill and Natasha said they have suppressed certain desires and goals throughout life because they didn't want to be ostracized for what they wanted. Long ago hurts left emotional residue.

The name calling (e.g. slut, whore, tomboy, dyke) heard in childhood may later become the name calling, words or actions of betrayal, or excluding behaviors that women use in adulthood. These behaviors reflect policing strategies that admonish or attempt to "get in line" women who have deviated from the narrowly defined gender behaviors and social roles proscribed for them. In fact, many women are afraid of standing up for women's rights for fear of being called pejorative names (feminist, feminist-nazi, "man-hater," lesbian) or other negative words used to put women down.

I (Erika) was getting a manicure when a reporter on television was discussing Rosie O'Donnell's departure from the television show *The View*. A woman seated next to me began cheering saying that it was about time she left as women should not be allowed to speak out in the way she did. I thought, "if Rosie were a man would this woman be so angry at her?" When girls and women deviate from what is deemed appropriate for female behavior, other women begin to turn on each other. Why would we do this to one other?

Something to Think About

> Was your behavior (words or actions) "policed" by your peers when you were in school? What did the other kids say to you? How were you treated? As an adult, have your actions been policed by other women? What happened?

In the United States, girls are socialized into culturally and socially defined categories of female behavior or femininity that is strict, narrow, and mutually exclusive from male behavior. A young girl is socialized at her earliest moments to think, feel, express, and behave in gender appropriate ways. By doing so, she unconsciously, unwittingly, and smoothly replicates the behaviors necessary to maintain strict gender roles. Depending on how seamlessly gender rules are transferred to her, she forms a strong gender identity as a female.

Young girls not only "police" themselves with regard to functioning in a gender appropriate manner, they also police their peers. Then they mature into adolescents and adult women who continue to police each other. Typically, any woman who thinks, talks, acts, or behaves outside these strictly defined gender behaviors may be seen as inferior, other, deviant, or less than a real female (e.g. lesbians). Surprisingly, women who are considered strikingly beautiful may also be policed and targeted by their peers.

From the standpoint of our current culture, there appears to be one and only one right way for a girl to grow up. Despite needs and desires to connect and belong, as a woman, she can end up being made to feel she is an outsider or deviant in multiple ways. She is an outsider to men because she is female, and if she is noticeably different, she can also be excluded and made to feel that she does not belong with other women. Many women keep girls and other women in line; they try and make the "deviant" ones behave the ways the culture suggests.

The net effect of living under a set of constricting double binds intertwined with strict gender rules and the experience of "working at" being female results in an emotional toll on a woman's sense of self and sense of well-being. Sandra Bem suggested that the gender rules alone can foster deep insecurity that evolves into a vicious cycle; a sense of insecurity based on a woman's experience of gender may be followed with internal conflict and followed again with more insecurity.[16]

The cost to the female self is exponential. Not only do women experience internal conflict and the sense of insecurity, women experience an almost unknowable and unspeakable self-hatred.

The difficulty? A woman lives with the absence of a congruent, authentic self. Absent an authentic self she is absent deep and enduring authentic connections. The thought of turning against (being angry with) men isn't possible. Instead she may turn on women because women represent that which she hates in herself, so it is much easier to hurt those who represent what she may not like in herself.

So where can she go or what can she do when she feels different or wants to be different? How can she act? What does she do with the feeling that she has no options, including expressing the feeling that she has no options? This situation is further complicated by social rules that constrain a woman's competence, anger, and difference. If she does authentically express herself, others policing her actions may result.

These are some of the reasons that underlie why women hurt, betray, backstab, trash-talk, or oppress other women. The cycle of self-hatred begins with: A girl is inferior from the start. She experiences several binds that constrict and confuse her. How she is socialized as a female further binds and further constricts her options for authentic self-expression. If she wants to express herself or do something about this situation, then she gets policed for it. She believes she has no place to turn, so she keeps everyone else in line and hurts them for being deviant or straying from the norm. It's the only power she has and can express—to turn on someone like herself.

Chapter VII

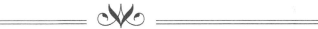

Oppressive Experiences

A woman's self concept develops through internalizing inter-actions with people in her social sphere, whether parents, teach-ers, friends, spouses, partners, girlfriends, boyfriends, peers, or col-leagues. Often she has relied on stereotypes of women to help her learn and define how she should behave.

A stereotype is a symbol for something else. It's a simplified way to generalize positive or negative attributes of an individual person or group, making it convenient and easy to categorize and label people or things. When there are a variety of characteristics that seem common to a number of individuals, especially if they are members of a particular group, then those same characteristics are often attributed to all people who are members of that group, whether the characteristics are true or not. Stereotypes become problematic, however, when these categories are used indiscrimi-nately, without fully considering a woman's unique attributes.

M. Heilman, a psychology researcher, suggested that gender stereotypes most likely play a key role in how women discriminate against other women. Implicit in these stereotypes are expecta-tions about how women should behave and what women are like; these can result in a woman's performance being devalued, her competence being penalized, or her successes denied.[1] Although competence, independence, ambition, and initiative are required for success, these qualities are still considered less desirable for women. Using derogatory terms against a successful woman ("bitch," "ice queen," "ball-buster," and "battle axe") is one way to devalue her sense of competence.[2]

Women who behave outside of conventional female stereotypes are seen as violating appropriate female behavior; consequently, they frequently elicit disapproval, negative reactions, or exclusion from desired groups or opportunities. When a woman is not aligned with a stereotypically feminine role the potential for hurtful behavior between women can occur.[3] One example includes female beauty pageant winners who acted outside their established norm by us-ing drugs, "flipping the bird," and videotaping sexually provocative behavior; they were later ostracized for their behavior by female peers.

Print and TV media have described the "mommy wars"—a situation where a group of women desiring careers ("career moms") have been pitted against a group of women desiring children and family (the "stay-at-home moms"). It often appears as if one group is right and the other wrong. These women are pressured into staking positions; they cannot comfortably have membership in either or both groups. Members of one group often then denigrate members of the other group.

Something to Think About

Consider all the different ways you identify yourself by thinking about all the groups to which you belong. They may include your cultural or ethnic affiliation, age, sex, religious or spiritual affiliation, whether you have a disability, or even your socioeconomic status. If you stop and think about it, you can probably come up with both positive and negative stereotypes that have been described for each of the different ways you identify yourself.

"In-Groups" and "Out-Groups"

We have a natural drive to develop meaningful relationships and be connected with others to satisfy a universal need to belong. We are part of groups to be close with people who are similar to us; what brings us together are things shared in common. Shared experiences and values create feelings of specialness and closeness. If others do not share the same history, qualities, abilities, and interests, groups can be harmful, especially to those who are not included.

Being deprived of satisfying opportunities to be included often results in feelings of anxiety, loneliness, depression, emotional distress, and even health problems. One of the strongest threats to *belonging* involves being socially excluded, and being excluded by groups to which you want to belong ranks among the most painful of human experiences.[4]

Something to Think About

Think about your different stages of life and the settings involved (e.g. elementary through high school, college, or various work settings). Were you in the "in-group" or the "out-group"? If you were not in the popular group, did you feel left out, like you didn't belong or fit in, were an outcast, or that there was something wrong with you? Were there groups that intentionally excluded you? Did you exclude others from your group(s)?

As with stereotypes, people tend to categorize themselves, and no matter how our social world is divided, on the basis of sex, skin color, ethnic group, socioeconomic status, occupation, or any other aspect, there will be a category to which a woman belongs. As she develops close relationships to women in her *in-group*, the more she and other *in-group* members tend to exclude women outside the group.[5]

Not only is a woman generally considered deviant and inferior if she is identified as belonging to some *out-group, out-group* members are also subjected to negative, harsh, or unfair treatment. For instance, any woman falling outside the stereotyped view of a woman (e.g. obese, aggressive, or manly looking) may experience harsh treatment from other women. Simply put, there are pressures from within and outside groups to behave in ways that match the female stereotype. It means a woman must accept and internalize characteristics attributed to stereotypically feminine women in U.S. culture, and then behave as she is "supposed to" behave.

The wildly popular MTV hit show The Hills centers around Lauren Conrad (LC) who is portrayed as the sweet, beautiful girl who is perfect and popular. Anyone in Lauren's circle is definitely part of the in-group. Initially, LC's best friend and roommate was Heidi Montag, but their friendship fell apart during the second season of the show when Montag began dating Spencer Pratt. By the season's end, Montag moved out of Lauren's apartment and in with Pratt. Since that time, the two girls have barely said a word to one another. They complete photo shoots separately and have them edited as if they appeared together. As a result of the broken friendship, Montag became a part of the out-group and was dubbed by many fans as the villain of the show. Their fight escalated when rumors began to spread that LC had made a sex tape with her ex-boyfriend, rumors that LC believes Montag and Pratt started. Perhaps Montag and Spencer created this rumor to seek revenge because they were kicked out of LC's in-group? Note that it was when Montag began dating Pratt that their friendship began to disintegrate.

In-groups and out-groups exist in every culture, and which groups are chosen to be in and out of favor may, of course, differ with regard to cultural differences, social status, gender, etc. To develop and sustain a sense of cohesion, group members frequently foster the experience of having a perceived common enemy. This sense of "us" and "them" helps create a sense of cohesion in a group, especially if the group members believe in their own superiority.

Subgrouping allows a woman to maintain stereotypes and dissociate herself from other women who she perceives as being unlike her, *often a first step to putting women down*. Subgrouping has already been observed among adolescent girls as they create their social groups by forming alliances and coalitions against other girls. Researcher Marjorie Goodwin found that adolescent school girls spend a bulk of their time making mean statements about other kids at school (including members of their own social group). They punished girls through cryptic comments and exchanges of collusive, knowing looks and gestures in the presence of the targeted individual; talk about her in her absence; exclude her from play, and yell insults from a distance.[6]

We have seen elements of subgrouping throughout the 2008 political season as fights on the show *The View* between staunch Republican Elizabeth Hasselback and Joy Behar, an equally committed Democrat, have at times devolved into these two women distancing from each other and occasionally putting the other down.

Status, Self-Hatred, and Hurtful Behavior

When there are high-status groups (men) and low-status groups (women, people of color), members of low-status groups often struggle to maintain a positive sense of self. Given this situation, women may attempt to move away from low-status groups by trying to "fit in" higher-status groups. An example of such behavior was displayed on *The Tyra Banks Show* (July 11, 2008), involving an episode on stereotypes associated with people's names. Near the end of the show, an African-American woman described how she had intentionally named her daughter Ashley, a Caucasian sounding name, in an effort to provide the greatest possible opportunities for her daughter. She believed that if she had given her child a more African sounding name, her daughter would have lost out on opportunities for advancement simply based on the name.

A woman has to deny aspects of herself to dissociate from her own in-group. Efforts to deny aspects of herself, dissociate from groups important to her, or behave in a manner that is not congruent with who she is are really manifestations of self-hatred . . . the underlying thread that leads women to hurt other women. On the basis of this self-hatred, a girl or woman lives up to (or down to) the expectations she thinks she can achieve.

Consider what is happening with the phenomenon of "reality TV." Reality TV or the American Idol or Talent Search series often offer the "average Jane" of society the chance to have a crack at both fame and fortune (perceived higher-status groups), thus leaving her lower-status groups behind. Clearly countless thousands are jumping at the chance to do just that. Or think about how many women attempt to model themselves after other women who are perceived to hold higher value in society (e.g. runway models, movie and TV stars, etc.), including putting themselves in debt or altering their bodies, just so they can be more like the higher-status group and less like the group to which they already belong.

Florence Kennedy (as cited in Paula Kaplan's book *Don't Blame Mother: Mending the Mother Daughter Relationship*) used the phrase "*horizontal hostility*" to describe this same situation, one in which members of the same oppressed, powerless, and marginalized group fight among and attack each other. You can also think of this as "in-fighting." [7] It is a form of prejudice exhibited by members of marginalized groups (as women are) against members of a similar marginalized group (other women). Women take out their feelings of anger, frustration, and mistrust on those who have equal or less power or status than they do. Not only do these attacks perpetuate victimization, they also divide women and prevent them from bonding and working together to tackle oppression. So women continue to hurt, betray, and backstab each other.

Trina, an African-American woman who attended one of our training workshops on women oppressing women, told us that because she was light-skinned in comparison to many of the other girls with whom she attended college, she was ridiculed and excluded from desired social activities. Even though the majority of the women in her social group at school were women of color, these women would shun her because she appeared "whiter" than them.

Internalized Sexism

Sexism is any mistreatment of women, including violence against women or women being objectified and treated as inferior. Any time a woman is devalued and treated other than as a respected human being, it is sexism. When a woman does not stand up for herself, tolerates abusive behavior from men, mistreats other women, or denies her own value as a woman, internalized sexism has occurred. It includes the negative feelings and/or self-hate that result from growing up in a sexist environment that devalues and denigrates women. It would not exist without the real external oppression found within our culture.

Women have internalized societal messages that undermine their self-worth, so achieving high self-esteem is difficult in a culture that devalues and trivializes women. When society devalues women, it creates the propensity for women to devalue each other, so it is not surprising that some women dislike and are hostile toward other women. Hostility toward other women can be viewed as self-hatred; accepting negative stereotypes and distrusting other women really is just a way of women rejecting themselves. When a woman devalues other women, she really devalues herself.

Phyllis Chesler, author of *Woman's Inhumanity to Woman*, believes that internalized sexism causes women to develop a double standard toward other women. Though women naturally seem to prefer joining together, they tend to suppress any real expression of jealousy, competitiveness, or aggressiveness based on fears of rupturing closeness or damaging friendship bonds. Instead women often resort to expressing hostility indirectly by manipulating and punishing targeted women through gossip, innuendo, and other forms of relationally hurtful behavior.[8]

Chapter VIII

Competition and Aggression

Socialized to be Sweet

Prior to the 1980s, researchers were only studying male aggressive behavior, and the notion of female aggression was practically non-existent. Authors such as Arnold Buss believed that aggression was solely a male phenomenon and he claimed that women were so rarely aggressive that female aggression wasn't even worth the trouble to study.[1]

Behavior differences between males and females are maintained by the messages girls and boys receive about how they "should be" in the world. Parents, media, and other societal influences encourage and reinforce traditional or stereotyped female behaviors such as shyness, fearfulness, niceness, goodness, quietness, and timidity in girls while discouraging females from displaying more stereotypical male behaviors such as aggressiveness and hostility.[2]

Girls learn from an early age that it is not acceptable to display overtly aggressive behaviors; they are socialized to avoid conflict, competition, and aggression, and instead are encouraged to create and maintain harmonious relationships. Girls as young as five years old understand sanctions against openly expressing their anger; as girls mature they internalize negative reactions others have to their anger.

Girls are taught to express their feelings, particularly angry or competitive feelings, quite differently than boys. Carol Gilligan, a Harvard researcher and scholar who is well known for her studies on girls and women, believes that girls tend to avoid competition and instead adopt the role of peacemaker, making efforts to diffuse conflict and preserve harmony within relationships.[3]

Most girls grow up experiencing double bind messages that prohibit them from asserting themselves, a bind that compromises good self-esteem and complicates overall healthy development. Girls are often fearful of living beyond the constricted roles into which they are socialized. In our society, as in most other cultures, assertive, aggressive, competitive, and independent behavior is valued and encouraged for males, not for females. Independent and assertive action is considered the domain of boys and men, consequently, girls do not typically learn how to effectively experience or express angry and competitive feelings.

Rachel Simmons, author of *Odd Girl Out*, notes that girls fear that expressing conflict will damage their relationships.[4] No question that girls and boys both experience anger, but because girls face so many rules and prohibitions against expressing anger they feel constrained from expressing themselves directly. Feeling such constraints, girls opt to withdraw or to express anger in more indirect ways. If direct expression is not sanctioned, then girls use relationally hurtful strategies as they mature into adult women.

Regardless of age, women frequently hold themselves in check. When women do express anger or exhibit competitive drive, they get categorized negatively, are often seen as deviant, and are demeaned further by being called a "bitch," "ball-buster," or lesbian. They are taught to so highly value close and intimate relationships that, sadly, women become very afraid of expressing angry or competitive feelings for fear that it will damage or ruin relationships. The truth is expressing anger is more real; women are more authentic when they do, and it not only strengthens them, it usually strengthens their relationships.

Competition and Meaner Women

At the most basic level, hurtful behavior between women occurs because of a woman's experience of inadequacy and self-hatred in the face of intense competition with other women. It develops over time and is influenced by various societal expectations, media influences, and biological and evolutionary pressures.

Women rarely talk openly about competition, yet they compete with each other to be the most beautiful, thinnest, and sexiest, generally for the most valued prize . . . a man. Women are not necessarily competing just for the man himself but for children she might conceive with him and for the other resources that he can provide (money, status, power, and prestige).

Author Leora Tanenbaum, *in her book Catfight, notes* that as many women compete for men, a result is that females develop self-hatred; girls and women devalue themselves and each other and then they may end up disassociating or disconnecting from other females.[5] To illustrate this point, see what the popular comedian Chris Rock said during his 2004 HBO standup comedy routine *Never Scared.*[6]

> "Women HATE women. You get any two girlfriends in this room, been girlfriends for twenty-five years, you put a man in between them . . . 'F–k that bitch,' 'F–k that bitch.' Guys are not like that. Guys actually think that there are other fish in the sea, and if a guy introduces his boy to his new girlfriend, and when they walk away, his boy goes, 'Aww man, she's nice, I gotta get me a girl like that.' If a woman introduces her new man to her girlfriend, and they walk away, her girlfriend goes, 'I gotta get HIM, and I will slit that bitch's throat to do it.' Every girl in here got a girlfriend they don't trust around their man."

So, we ask, is Chris Rock right? Do women *really* hate women?

We really believe that women don't hate women. Women speak freely and comfortably about needing each other and are known to have great loving and supportive friendships. Close-knit groups of female friends are the norm. The reality is, however, that women do compete against each other, and do hurt each other. Film, television, radio, and the Internet have all been used to sensationalize hostility between women.

Think of how media and marketing efforts play up and intentionally create competition between women, as opposed to recognizing and enjoying the diversity women bring to friendships. For instance, the sole focus of the brief "reality" show *Age of Love* was to have women in their forties compete against women in their twenties . . . all for one man's affection. Another example involves the competition between the stay-at-home mom and the career woman. This particular competition has been escalated further with media-driven "mommy wars" demanding to know . . . who is the better woman? When women's personal choices are polarized in these ways, it seems inevitable for women to fail. There is no domain between women that remains untouched. Women even compete with each other over attractiveness by surgically altering body size and body parts.

Unquestionably, the demands for girls and women have changed over the past fifty to one hundred years. Girls and women today experience much more pressure than their mothers and grandmothers. At that time, women largely filled the role of chief nurturer and caretaker of children and home. Author Susan Shapiro Barash in *Tripping the Prom Queen: The Truth about Women and Rivalry*, writes that one of the chief reasons women engage in female-to-female competition is due to the difficulties females face trying to get ahead in today's society. She notes that it doesn't matter whether women compete for men, a successful career, or to remain eternally youthful and beautiful, it seems clear that the glass ceiling and the unrealistic standards for female beauty still exist. When a woman looks at other women who appear to have succeeded where she thinks she has failed, the pain can feel almost intolerable.[7]

Dr. Deborah Cox and her colleagues have been studying this particular issue—the "beauty culture"—specifically the competition between women involving issues of beauty, including competition between mothers and daughters. They suggest that beauty translates into power and privilege, yet it is defined in ways that are impossible to maintain. As Dr. Cox notes, women's "code of silence" about these issues "leaves us alienated from each other, resulting in mistrust, isolation, fear of being outdone, compared, or abandoned."[8]

As if competition isn't already fierce enough around beauty, Dr. Cox describes how part of the competition is to appear the most non-competitive or the most unconcerned about beauty.

> It's confusing . . . how does one appear non-competitive and be intensely competitive at the same time?! The competition between women around beauty also goes way beyond just attractiveness or good looks. The competition also involves relationship success, career status, prestige, wealth, a good family life, children, etc.[9]

Others, such as author Leora Tannenbaum, believe that females compete with one another as a result of confusing and often contradictory messages about gender role expectations. She describes hostile behavior between women as a coping and frustration-venting mechanism, a response to insecurities about failing to live up to unrealistically high standards.[10]

Though improving, women live in a culture that belittles, devalues, and discredits them; having learned their social place and value and having experienced oppression (whether conscious of it or not), women learn to take out anger and aggression on other similarly oppressed women. It feels easier, safer, and less dangerous to attack each other than to attack the source of the problem.

And now women compete for everything; the competition goes well beyond being able to "get a man." The pressure has, in fact, greatly intensified. *Women no longer only compete for men, they also compete against men and against women* for career positions, financial success, status, power, and prestige. Women compete with each other for all of these achievements and resources. Countless societal pressures demand women to "be all" and "do it all." The more difficult it feels for women to gain access to these resources, the more likely women are to hurt each other.

Chapter IX

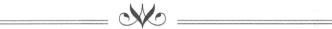

Building Collaborative Relationships
and Community

Bonds not Binds:
Creating Positive Connections with Women

Perhaps you have already explored thoughts and feelings about your identity as a woman; comfort and desire to bond with women in your life; relationships with your daughters; girls you are mentoring; and female acquaintances or women who you count as close friends. For those who have not, we would like to see you experience a strong sense of self and closer, more supportive relationships with the women in your life.

If you have great female friends and are close with and surrounded by a group of supportive, loving women . . . that's great! Cherish these women, nurture the friendships, and celebrate what you have fostered for yourself. Make sure to consciously set aside a regular time to talk or meet. Create rituals that honor your time together. Establish a "girls' night out" that is a routine part of your schedule. Appreciate and nurture your friendships. The sense of community you create is essential to your overall health. Breaking a tie between close friends may lead to giving up more than just having contact with that once close friend. There can be long-term negative consequences that influence health and emotional well-being.

Several studies emphasize the importance of and need for friendship and companionship as an essential element of well-being. Results from a landmark study conducted by Harvard Medical School about social networks and healthy aging found that **maintaining close friendships is just as important to overall health as not smoking, eating a nutritional diet, and exercising on a regular basis**. Close friends contribute to living a longer, healthier life. The more friends one has and the more time spent with them, the higher one's level of functioning.[1]

Making Changes

Throughout life, a woman receives innumerable subtle and blatant messages about how she should function in the world. Women must no longer be defined by such messages. Change, if desired, takes time. True change is incremental. A woman can be assertive, speak her mind, express her anger, determine her path, compete for what she wants to achieve, and be exuberant and passionate in its pursuit.

If you raise or mentor a girl, be proactive in educating her to understand the world around her. Help her decipher, sort through, and challenge gender stereotypes and gender messages she receives and accepts as fact. She needs to seriously consider what she is being asked *to do* or who she is being asked *to be.* Start as early as possible in her life to address issues that allow her to make more conscious choices about the woman she would like to be in the world.

And if you are a young or adolescent girl, well then . . . lucky you! Make thoughtful choices along the way. Dream your dreams and be in charge of your life in many ways that women before you may have not. You have important choices to make and challenges to face. You have to start by thinking about what you really want for yourself. Keep in mind what Lyn Mikel Brown, in her book *Girlfighting,* said about friendships with other girls.

> "Girls' friendships with other girls, as wonderful as they can be and as important as they are, will be measured time and again against two prevailing ideals—being like boys or being liked by boys; being girls who do what boys do or being girls boys want. As these two culturally sanctioned choices become more defined and encouraged, betrayal and competition, rejection and exclusion will be focused on those girls who challenge these pathways or threaten a girl's status and power by being a better, more successful traveler on one road or another."[2]

Self-Reflection and Self-Repair

Take some time to reflect on your relationships. Your first step, either as an adolescent girl or as a woman, is to take a close look at your experiences with girls as you grew up through childhood and adolescence and what your friendships with women have generally been up till now. The act of self-reflection leads to awareness and awareness can lead to change. It's a gift to yourself to take yourself, and what you truly deserve, seriously. Allow yourself time to consider the questions that are provided for you in *Appendix A*. Journal if you wish.

Regardless of age, if you desire changes in your relationships with women, you can "start wherever you are." Understand how you have related to females in your life. Who were you in those relationships? How did you feel? How were you treated? How did you behave? Can you identify any particular patterns with girls when you were young or with women as you have matured? Is there any particular issue or theme that emerges?

Hurting Others Now?

If you are a woman who has treated other women in ways that betray, exclude, demean, or devalue them, please pause and reflect before you behave in hurtful ways in the future. What purpose do you want to achieve by hurting another? Are you feeling competitive with other women, and if so, for what prize? Can you express your anger or competitiveness in a manner that is more direct and respectful of the woman or women toward whom you have these feelings? Are there other means by which you can access what you want? How can you achieve what you want collaboratively? Are you allowing your children to express anger you yourself have not yet expressed?

Consider reaching out to women you have hurt and offer a sincere apology and interest in repairing the strained or damaged relationship. If you are still hurting other women, take a closer look at yourself, perhaps consider getting professional help, and make a commitment to stop hurting others.

Attacking behavior between women is often tied to experiences of betrayal and distrust, so please consider the source of your betrayal and distrust. How have you been affected? How have girls and women broken your trust or betrayed you? Any attack on another woman ultimately is an act of self-hatred and a symbolic attack on yourself.

Why the need to reflect on these questions? Why go back and, in essence, relive some of that pain or look more closely at the pain you may be experiencing now? When emotional injuries go unaddressed, then people find ways to create a life around the pain, mostly to protect themselves from the initial emotional pain or any other emotional wound resembling it. The result? People cut off aspects of themselves from others . . . particularly female friends. Read about one woman who tried to cut herself off from early childhood pain.

In one of the workshops, a woman in her late twenties described how she was realizing in that moment that she was one of the "mean girls" when she was young. She said she only had close male friends and not only did she have no close female friends, she didn't like women. As she continued to talk, she recalled very hurtful experiences with her sister and other girls when she was young. She was in tears as she described how she had only allowed herself to be close to boys and men because of her early hurtful experiences, and that she treated girls meanly so she herself would not be hurt. As a young girl she promised herself and was emphatic about never letting anyone have the "upper hand"; she didn't want anyone to doubt who had the power and control. More tears flowed as she acknowledged how much she must have missed out on.

Repairing Emotional Ruptures

Why deal with these early emotional wounds and scars? If you don't, as an adult you are more likely to treat other women in a hurtful manner or you are at risk of vicariously living your hurt and anger through your daughter(s) as they act aggressively or hurtfully toward their own peers. So if you are a mother, caretaker, mentor, or role model and have responsibilities for raising or mentoring girls, take some time to reflect on your experiences.

Healing and change start when you become aware of damaged relationships with women in your life; missed opportunities for genuine friendship or closeness with women, personal growth, or for professional advancement (promotions, more responsibility); and loss of self-respect from how you have been treated or for how you have treated other women.

If you have been the target of women's hurtful behavior, similar to the woman above, perhaps you have also said, "I won't let anyone get that close to me ever again." If you have, you too risk losing your aliveness and vitality and the benefits of close friendship that you so richly deserve. Grieving can open the space to get close to others again. If you allow yourself to be aware of these losses and to truly grieve them, then, through grieving, it is much more likely you will feel motivated to "be" and act in the world with a greater sense of initiative and confidence. We think you will be much more interested in being who you truly are.

Grief involves feelings that can range from intense rage to profound sadness (and all the feelings in between). It means looking at opportunities or goals that perhaps were never made available to you nor realized by you. It means thinking about how you treated and how you were treated by others in childhood or as a teenage girl and the impact that behavior had upon you, perhaps invisible wounds with indistinguishable scars that are now really worth looking at. And once you have looked back and understood the lessons your experience can bring, forgiveness is the next step. Forgiving others and forgiving yourself.

Tips for Mending, Tending, and Befriending

Making sense of life experience helps people lead more effectively, so whether you are in a mothering or a mentoring role, it's important to take a close look at your life and how you behave toward and are treated by female friends, peers, sisters, colleagues, co-workers, supervisors, or parents. You serve as the best model for your daughter to learn how to be a loving and compassionate person. Lead with your compassion. Don't try to follow what she does so you can be a "cool" mom. Believe it or not, parents lose credibility when they behave this way. Your daughter will closely observe everything you do in life; along with clothing, food, money, dating, marriage, work, friends, or self-discipline, she will notice how you handle your feelings and express yourself.

Model Appropriate Expression of Anger

Women seem much more adept at handling sad and vulnerable feelings that they tend to turn inward, as opposed to angry and competitive feelings, which are outwardly expressed. As women learn to tolerate, manage and directly express unpleasant feelings of anger, aggression, competitiveness, envy, jealousy or hurt more effectively with each other, we will see less relationally hurtful behavior between women. Instead, women will create genuine connections that are dynamic and vitally alive. So, feel it, say it, don't belabor it, let it go.

Model appropriate use of anger and direct expression of it within your relationships and it can help girls understand more about how to handle their angry feelings. It can also help girls understand that conflicts naturally occur in friendships and that these conflicts can be resolved in a direct and loving manner without damaging the friendship. Help your child articulate painful feelings—she may have to go through the messiness of learning how to get the words out—even if it is uncomfortable.

Start Young

Socialization of girls starts the moment she is born. Actually, it can start in utero, including the moment parents know the child's sex. Girls must be made aware of the subtle and not-so-subtle influences on what they are being asked to value, how they behave, what they aspire to, and who they are encouraged to become. To these ends, girls must be made aware of and taught to think critically about all the different ways they can be influenced in their lives. Awareness leads to greater choice, even in youth and adolescence.

With the anticipated conflicts that occur as a child ages, you can help provide your daughter an opportunity to practice handling unpleasant feelings and difficult conflicts simultaneously. It is crucial that a girl learn to manage (tolerate) unpleasant and uncomfortable feelings. Once she has achieved relative comfort or success doing so, then it's important to teach her how to more directly and effectively express angry or competitive feelings. Learning constructive responses to these feelings can prevent destructive expressions of anger (e.g. self-mutilation, eating disorders, and drug use). Girls must also learn that revenge is not the proper response to an experience of having been "wronged."

Address Hurtful Behavior Between Girls and Between Women

You will have multiple opportunities to observe women oppress women or girls be hurtful and hostile with friends and peers. Perhaps you can stop the behavior when it occurs between your friends. The incidents between children (and there will be many) create opportunities to talk openly and forthrightly with girls about "girlfighting." Using discretion, confront the behaviors when they occur. These are times to talk with girls about how relationships work and how they can build friendships that are enduring and authentic. Talk about how conflicts are a natural part of relationships, that all relationships involve learning to manage uncomfortable or unpleasant feelings (most notably feelings of anger, disappointment, jealousy, sadness), and that the healthiest and most effective means to creating authentic and enduring relationships is to tell the truth within them. Girls must be taught to express such feelings in a compassionate and direct manner, as opposed to engaging in undercutting, undermining, and hurtful behaviors.

Stopping mean behavior does not mean stopping anger. Whatever your role, you need to tolerate and be responsive to the anger you witness or hear. If anger is the only response she has, help her identify and be in touch with the issues and hurt hiding underneath her anger. There may be important concerns to address. If her anger seems appropriate to the situation but her aggressive response is not (or she has been a target of such aggression), then this is a perfect opportunity to help her effectively express feelings of anger.

Lyn Mikel Brown suggests engaging girls' anger, as this anger is about self-respect and indicates a girl is taking herself seriously; using it in relationally aggressive ways is really about displaced anger. It can also help her develop a sense of fairness and justice.[3] And if you observe hurtful and hostile behavior, use these opportunities to model respect and caring and to address important issues (e.g. how to stand up for herself, expectations of friendships, gender roles).[4]

Generally "mean girls" and "mean women" are ridiculed and isolated. Think about and talk about both sides of the situation—who is/was the aggressor and who is/was being hurt.[5] Why were mean or excluding behaviors chosen as the means for dealing with the situation? Go after the deeper issues involved with meanness as a strategy for problem solving and the cost to relationships and authenticity.

Finally, challenge and confront the angry and aggressive behaviors that girls and women turn inward. If you observe signs that suggest girls are behaving in directly self-destructive behaviors (e.g. eating disorders, self-mutilation), understand that these actions represent anger and aggression turned inward. They are acts steeped in self-hatred. If you teach or mentor girls in any capacity, you are in a perfect position to talk with girls about these issues.

Exposing and Responding to Societal and Cultural Influences

A woman is constantly barraged with countless messages, influences, and demands to fit into a stereotyped female role. She can cultivate the ability to see behind these messages, to develop a sort of "double vision" so she can more effectively understand, choose, or reject the double messages and standards by which she is asked to live. Having double vision means she understands both the superficial and the complex, nuanced deeper meanings of any message. She can start by being aware of how she has followed traditional female stereotypes and critically consider what to keep or change. She should do what she loves and what works for her so she enjoys who she is. A woman should envision what she wants for herself regardless of traditional or stereotypic gender roles and make choices that are the most congruent for her.

Explode Gender Choices
Broaden the definition of what it means to be female to encompass all the various ways femininity can be expressed in our culture now. Rather than having one strict, constraining view of femininity,

think of women as having "femininities" so that women have many choices on how they can express themselves in the world. Move past rigid "either-or" type of thinking that a woman either fits into a traditional female role or she does not. Women who are "do-ers," independent, assertive, achievement-oriented, athletic, lesbian, or transgender also need to be valued. Consider the type of women you want included in your social support network. Do these women fit or follow traditional stereotypes of the female gender role or are their experiences more gender diverse?

Respond to Double Binds

"Double vision" can also help you decipher and respond to hidden double bind messages. First, simply recognize that they exist. Second, act on your awareness. Recognize that you have *choices* about how to behave. You can challenge double binds by speaking with other women about what you experience so you don't feel alone.

Express yourself. Take a stand. Step beyond the mold you are being asked to fit and instead actively pursue your dreams and aspirations with less emphasis on what (you think) others think of you and more emphasis on what you think of yourself and who you want to be in the world. The binds will only constrict you—what you say and how you behave. You must be willing to take risks to go beyond these constrictions so you can more authentically be yourself.

Kathleen Jamieson, in her book *Women and Double Binds*, describes eight steps for responding to double binds. Her suggestions include: a) *reframing* (seeing the double bind options as false), b) *recovering* (understanding the history of women's lives and the progress women have made), c) *reclaiming language* (not identifying as a victim), d) *recasting language* (turning negative labels into positive identifiers or assets; e.g. "behind every man is a woman in the house . . . and senate"), e) *identifying equal opportunity alternatives* (e.g. himbo vs. bimbo), f) *rewriting material* (e.g. changing religious liturgy to include women), g) *telling your own narrative,* and h) *confounding the stereotypes* (e.g. being a bright, competent, well-liked, assertive, attractive woman).[6]

Anger and Competition: What to Do?

We live in a much more competitive society, and our world now requires skills to function and thrive in this competitive environment. Boys and men tend to have many more outlets for learning how to manage aggressive and competitive impulses. Authors generally agree that one way boys learn how to manage their anger and competitive feelings occurs through playing team and organized sports. In the ideal, they learn to suppress their desire to be hurtful toward others by channeling this energy into sports activities.

Increase girls' participation in competitive and team sports. Girls and women can have the same experience as boys and men do—that they can compete (perhaps even fiercely) on the field or on the court with each other as competitors, yet walk off the field as friends. Engaging in intense competition can also help girls and women develop more effective strategies for tolerating and managing the experience of anger or aggression, feelings that they often do not tolerate well. Healthy competition between them does not lessen the connection they can have with each other.

While team sports and similar activities are much more available to girls now, consider how your community can create more opportunities for girls to engage in athletic, sport, and team activities more generally and competitive and team sports (e.g. soccer, basketball) more specifically. Re-instituting mandatory physical education requirements from elementary through high school could be beneficial for girls.

Think of the human body as a metaphor for emotional well-being. When girls and women engage in activities to develop physical strength, it can help them experience a greater sense of their own emotional strength and confidence. When they engage in physical activity (especially a martial arts activity), they learn how to "own" their space, both literally and figuratively "taking a stand." If a girl or woman is able to rely on her body, it can help her develop the parallel emotional experience of believing that she can rely on herself and "stand her own ground."[7]

Be Technologically Savvy and Media Literate

We have had conversations with several experts who discuss the use and effects of technology and media in our culture. The trends are clear and many are not positive. Some technology use compromises our ability to create and sustain genuine human loving connections. There are many stories of women sitting right next to each other, and rather than turning to one another to talk, they were "texting" each other on their cell phones! Or texting at length while out socially with others.

Consider how you use technology. Are you using it to support and nurture your relationships with women and create community, in ways that compromise your connections with them (e.g. take away from face-to-face contact, decrease available time together), or in ways that hurt them (e.g. invade privacy, gossip, betray, tarnish reputations)?

Become Media Literate
Learn to critique the messages to which you are almost endlessly exposed, whether through television, film, radio, print, or

through advertising (in all media venues). This requires becoming media literate. Dr. Jean Kilbourne, a well-known media expert, emphasized on our Women's Inspiration radio show that media literacy is a necessary next step if we are to change our culture into one that is more sensitive and responsive to not only women, but also men and people of color.[8]

What is *media literacy?* The *New Mexico Media Literacy Project* (www.nmmlp.org) describes media literacy as the ability to critically consume (watch, read, or listen) and create media. Goals include providing the necessary knowledge/education and critical thinking skills or strategies to access, analyze, evaluate, and produce media.[9]

Become an informed consumer. When girls and women are media literate, they can more effectively decipher the complex messages received from all forms of media (e.g. TV, radio, recorded music, Internet, newspapers, magazines, books, videos/DVDs, video games, games and toys and other media, marketing through TV ads, billboards and other signage, and packaging). Such knowledge can help them discern how their time, energy and money are spent. These skills can be taught in school, clubs, parent organizations (e.g. parent-teacher associations or parenting skills training groups), or several other related community organizations.

Media literacy helps girls and women understand the obvious (or superficial content) of each media message and the less obvious messages and meanings (the subtext) that are hidden beneath the surface. It helps them create their own media messages, with an understanding of the meanings they seek to convey. Drawing directly from *The New Mexico Media Literacy Project*, here is a sampling of some of the media skills one can develop, regardless of age:[10]

1. Understand how media messages create meaning
2. Identify who created a particular media message
3. Recognize what the media maker wants us to believe or do
4. Name the "tools of persuasion" used

5. Recognize bias, spin, misinformation, and lies
6. Discover the part of the story that's not being told
7. Evaluate media messages based on your own experiences, beliefs, and values
8. Create and distribute your own media messages
9. Become advocates for change in our media system

Learn what to watch for and critically analyze the messages conveyed by all different forms of media (e.g. commercials, TV episodes, comedies, talk shows, movies, dramas, etc.). Use "double vision" to decipher the messages, both overt and covert, that suggest what women's roles are and how women should relate with other women, and how women should relate to men.

Learn how to watch and listen with critical eyes and ears. Whether it is on radio (from Ryan Seacrest to Rush Limbaugh to Howard Stern to National Public Radio or Pacifica Radio), or on film, look and listen for the deeper messages. First, take time to think about your own viewing and listening patterns . . . what do you watch? Who do you listen to? Second, pay attention to the issues or content on which they commonly focus. What consistent themes do they address? Who supports their programming? What do they want you to believe or buy? Third, be less emotionally involved as you watch or listen to the program; be less invested in each of the character's lives.[11] Step back. See some of the programs like the *Bad Girls Club* more as a situation comedy. Lastly, think about it . . . are these girls and women people you truly want to emulate? What messages are they conveying about women?

Several organizations exist now that monitor media content more actively and closely. Media Watch, for example, started in 1984 with a mission of helping create more informed consumers of mass media by distributing media literacy information through a variety of venues. Their purpose is to challenge abusive stereotypes and other biased images commonly found in the media. Their efforts include exposing situations where there is an attempt to silence marginalized groups (e.g. women and people of color).

See Appendix B for The Center for Media Literacy's Five Key Questions for evaluating media and Appendix C for other media literacy websites and related information.

Be an Activist

Taking action helps people heal. Perhaps you found something here that inspires you to change your life, relationships, or community. You can be an *advocate* or an *activist* for women's well-being. Many public agencies and corporations have instituted policies to prevent hostile work environments. If no policy is in effect, you can be instrumental in initiating and supporting a "*zero tolerance*" policy addressing oppressive behaviors that occur at your work site or in organizations to which you belong. This approach entails educating individuals in the organization about what is considered acceptable behavior.

Policy changes can also involve *media oversight,* especially regarding gender stereotypic, inequitable, highly sexualized, aggressive, and violent content. You can engage in *media activism.* Think more about what you read, watch, and listen to. Contact corporations whose products you buy or the media outlets that serve you and convey your opinion and view of their advertising and programming content.

Join established organizations where others are already engaged in changing the media environment. Privately or publicly engage in boycotting activities or corporations that demean women. Create opportunities for girls and women to join together to work collaboratively for a cause or mission larger than themselves. It is important for more voices to be heard.

Control your media environment by being more selective about what you read, listen to, or watch, in a manner similar to being selective about what friends you choose to hang out with. Actively choose how much you will use technology in your life and decrease your involvement with technology and media by cutting down on time spent on the Internet, watching TV (see www.turnoffyourtv.com), listening to music, or reading the newspaper and magazines. Instead get more involved with your kids, partner, spouse, and friends in physical or social activities.

Children who observe and become desensitized to hurtful, hateful, or violent behavior grow up to be adults who may be less sensitized to such behavior, and then they can become the same adults who are hurtful to others. Dr. Craig Anderson described brain research which suggests that negative effects of video violence can be seen in twenty minutes in the brain.[12] Think of what hours, days, weeks, and years are doing to your children! If you are interested, one good starting place is learn about the work of Dr. Craig Anderson and his colleagues on the effects of media violence on kids in his book, *Violent Video Game Effects on Children and Adolescents: Theory, Research, and Public Policy*.[13]

Act with Integrity

The primary reason for writing this book was to understand why women hurt, betray, backstab, or trash-talk other women. We know that the experience of self-hatred in the face of a highly competitive and oppressive culture is a central thread underlying this hurtful behavior. A second reason for writing this book was to help women reclaim their lives so that they can feel the freedom to be the women they desire to be—not fitting into someone else's cookie cutter mold and not feeling like they "just had to" fit into society's stereotypical view of women.

To the degree that you have made sense of your own experience and choices and have clarity on where you are going, we are genuinely pleased for you. As you move forward, we want you to have the kinds of experiences where you feel your talents abilities, personality, and worth *are* valued by those individuals who people your life . . . in other words, to be fully visible to others.

Understand that any comment or act that oppresses another woman chips away and erodes a woman's self-esteem, integrity, and sense of self. Respond to women in a manner that supports their integrity—experiences where they receive recognition or appropriate acknowledgement, feel emotionally satisfied or gratified from exchanges with others, feel a sense of worth and legitimacy, feel personally validated from contact with others absent confusion about what the experience or exchange meant, feel respected overall as an individual, and feel a sense of dignity and a solid sense of identity.[14]

Appendix A

Your Female Relationships

As a girl:

What did you think about the girls around you?

Did you compete with other girls? What were you competing for?

How were you treated by girls as you grew up?

How did you treat other girls? What did you do?

How would you have liked to have behaved?

If you treated anyone hurtfully, do you notice any pattern to who you treated poorly and why? What would you have done differently?

Were you in one or more cliques?

What did these cliques represent for you?

Who (really) defined your choices?

What did you like about your friendships with girls?

As a woman:

How do you see yourself now?

What do you like about your friendships with women?

How would you like them to be different now?

Do you compete with other women?

What are you competing for?

How do you currently treat women?

How are you treated by other women?

Are you who you want to be in this world today?

Who (really) defines your choices?

What obstacles / challenges must be confronted for you to achieve all you aspire to be and to do?

The Message and the Messengers

Were you socialized a particular way as you grew up?

Who was influencing you?

What role did your parents or caretakers have?

What role did teachers or mentors have?

What role did your peers have?

What role did the variety of print, TV, and film influences have
on your choices?

Did you fit the stereotype of a conventional female?

Were you trying to fit that specific role because it felt right to
you, or were you primarily socialized into it?

Appendix B

Center for Media Literacy

Five Key Questions for Evaluating Media

1. Who created this message?
2. What creative techniques are used to attract my attention?
3. How might different people understand this message differently?
4. What values, lifestyles, and points of view are represented in or omitted from this message?
5. Why is this message being sent?

Five Key Questions to evaluate media as you read, watch, or listen.[12]

(www.medialit.org, 2002–2007)

Appendix C

Media Literacy Resources

There is a lot of information available and many more websites than we have listed here. As a place to start, check out these websites for more information:

Center for Media Literacy	www.medialit.org
Geena Davis Institute for Media Literacy	www.thegeenadavisinstitute.org
The New Mexico Media Literacy Project	www.nmmlp.org
American Psychological Association	www.apa.org/pi/wpo/sexualization.html
Media Literacy	www.medialiteracy.com
Media Literacy Clearinghouse	www.frankwbaker.com
Understand Media	www.understandmedia.com
Media Education Foundation	www.mediaed.org
National Assoc. for Media Literacy Education	www.amlainfo.org/home
Hardy Girls, Healthy Women	www.hardygirlshealthywomen.org/index.php
New Moon Girl Media	www.newmooncatalog.com
Jean Kilbourne	www.jeankilbourne.com
Girls Incorporated	www.girlsinc.org
Dads and Daughters	www.dadsanddaughters.org/home/index.html
Women's Media Center	www.womensmediacenter.com
Third Wave Foundation	www.thirdwavefoundation.org
Words Can Work	www.wordscanwork.com
Girls, Women + Media Project	www.mediaandwomen.org/resources

(a great link to a variety of other websites and resources)

Appendix D

Women Oppressing Women: The Pathway Explained

Women hurt, betray, backstab, and trash-talk other women on the basis of a complex interplay of factors, including brain biology, evolutionary, media, double binds, gender, group behavior, and oppressive influences. Women behave these ways toward each other essentially on the basis of self-hatred—a self-hatred borne out of an experience of being considered inferior from birth, intertwined with culture's gender socialization practices (which includes all the double-bind, gender, and unrelenting media messages) and all other means by which girls can be influenced (parents, teachers, religious practices, peers, etc.).

From birth, women are faced with the experience of either being seen as inferior or being made to feel as if they are inferior. Women continue to live in a male-centered culture and despite countless other opportunities available to women, largely they continue to be socialized into rigid gender roles, most commonly that of a stereotypically feminine woman. Though not necessarily conscious to women, these act as oppressive forces against them.

Women come to accept these elements as fact, so that anyone that deviates from these norms is even more inferior and seen as a "fair" target (whether conscious or not); women seem quick to chastise, be hostile to, diminish, denigrate, deride, betray, backstab, trash-talk, or exclude a woman who lives outside these norms. Women who are more stereotypically feminine and fit the norm are the females that most women more directly compete with, again, perhaps in ways that are not fully conscious to them. Their competitive drive and the way they compete (relationally vs. physically aggressive) is linked to evolutionary influences and early caretaking roles, competing first and foremost with each other for a man and all the resources he can bring (including food, shelter, childen). Given changes in culture and changes in women's ensuing roles (return to the work force), women now also compete against men and against women for career positions, status, prestige, financial resources, and more.

By and large, women have not been taught how to experience or express angry or competitive feelings very effectively. So females use meanness as a coping strategy in and of itself. And experiences of ongoing oppression eventually lead to effects of oppression (self-hate, emotional numbing/cut-off, rage, silence and shame, social isolation); more experiences of oppression generally either give way to giving up or being hurtful to others. Once oppressed, a woman feels stripped of her personal integrity. As a result, she may feel lost or invisible, which just keeps the cycle going.

Women oppress women because of the self-hatred that comes from subordinating needs, wants, desires, and expressions of competition, anger, aggression, and a woman's true self. Women desire respect and recognition, experiencing and expressing genuine personal power, having trusting and authentic relationships, and living with integrity. These desires are difficult to accomplish when a woman's authentic self has been and is denied.

NOTES

CHAPTER I: INTRODUCTION

[1] Yomtobian, E. (2005). *A theoretical model of women oppressing women: Contextual factors, psychological processes and the developmental trajectory.* Unpublished doctoral thesis, Phillips Graduate Institute, Encino, CA.

[2] Jost, J. (1997). An experimental replication of the depressed-entitlement effect among women. *Psychology of Women Quarterly, 21,* 387–393.

[3] Chesler, P. (2002). *Woman's inhumanity to woman.* Nation Books: NY.

CHAPTER II: SMACKDOWN!

[1] Fey, T. (Screenplay), & Waters, M. (Director). (2004). *Mean girls* [Motion picture]. United States: Paramount Pictures

2   Wiseman, R. (2002). *Queen bees and wannabees: Helping your daughter survive cliques, gossip, boyfriends, and other realities of adolescence.* New York: Crown Publishers.

[3] Lutz, K. M., & Smith, K. (Screenplay) & Wolf, F. (Director). (2008). *The house bunny* [Motion Picture]. United States: Happy Madison Productions.

[4] Björkqvist, K. & Osterman, K., Lagerspetz, K. M. J., Landau, S. F., Caprara, G. V., & Fraczek, A. (2001). Aggression, victimization, and sociometric status: Findings from Finland, Israel, Italy, and Poland (p.113). In M. Ramirez & D. S. Richardson, (Eds.), *Cross-cultural approaches to research on aggression and reconciliation* (p. 111–119). Huntington, NY: Nova Science Publishers.

[5] Underwood, M. K. (2003). *Social aggression among girls.* New York: Guilford Press.

[6] Galen, B. R., & Underwood, M. K. (1997). A developmental investigation of social aggression among children. *Developmental Psychology, 33,* 589–600.

7   Crick, N. R., & Grotpeter, J. K. (1995). Relational aggression, gender, and social-psychological adjustment. *Child Development, 66,* 710–722.

8   Galen, B. R., & Underwood, M. K. (1997). A developmental investigation of social aggression among children. *Developmental Psychology, 33,* 589–600.

9   National Crime Prevention Council. (2003). Bullying, not terrorist attack, biggest threat seen by U.S. teens. Washington, DC: (press release).

10 Wiredsafety.org – *The world's largest internet safety and help group* (n.d.). Retrieved July 13, 2008 from http://wiredsafety.org/

11 Chu, J. (2005). You wanna take this online? Cyberspace is the 21st century bully's playgroup where girls play rougher than boys. *Time,* Vol. 166, 6.

12 Simmons, R. (2002). *Odd girl out: The hidden culture of girl's aggression.* NY: Harcourt Brace.

13 Gray, K. (2006). *How mean can teens be? "Primetime" special shows how the internet can fuel bullying and fighting.* Retrieved October 12, 2006, from http://abcnews.go.com/Primetime/story?id=2421562&page=1

14 Celizic, M. (2008). *Teens videotape beating as revenge for online posts.* Retrieved June 2, 2008, from http://www.msnbc.msn.com/id/24009077/

15 Conway, A. (2005). Girls, aggression, and emotion regulation. *American Journal of Orthopsychiatry, 75,* 2.

16 Conway, A. (2005). Girls, aggression, and emotion regulation. *American Journal of Orthopsychiatry, 75,* 2.

17 Conway, A. (2005). Girls, aggression, and emotion regulation. *American Journal of Orthopsychiatry, 75,* 2.

18 Lamb, S. (2002). *The secret lives of girls: What good girls really do–sex play, aggression, and their guilt.* The Free Press (Simon and Schuster): NY.

19 Lamb, S. (2002). *The secret lives of girls: What good girls really*

do–sex play, aggression, and their guilt. The Free Press (Simon and Schuster): NY.

[20] Casey-Cannon, S., Hayward, C., & Gowen, K. (2001). Middle-school girl's reports of peer victimization: Concerns, consequences, and implications. *Professional School Counseling, 5,* 138–144.

[21] Crick, N. R., & Grotpeter, J. K. (1996). Children's treatment by peers: Victims of relational and overt aggression. *Development and Psychopathology, 8,* 367–380.

[22] Ladd, B. K., & Ladd, G. W. (2001). *Variations in peer victimization: Relations in peer maladjustment.* In J. Juvonen & S. Graham (Eds.), Peer harassment in school: The plight of the vulnerable and victimized (p. 25–48). New York: Guildford Press.

[23] Simmons, R. (2002). *Odd girl out: The hidden culture of girl's aggression.* NY: Harcourt Brace.

CHAPTER III: THE FEMALE BRAIN: WIRED FOR HURT

[1] Baron-Cohen, S. (2003). *The essential difference: The truth about the male and female brain.* New York: Basic Books.

[2] Siegel, D. J. (1999). *The developing mind: Toward a neurobiology of interpersonal experience.* New York: The Guilford Press.

[3] Siegel, D. J. (2007). *The mindful brain: Reflection and attunement in the cultivation of well-being.* New York: W.W. Norton & Company.

[4] Schore, A. (2003). *Affect regulation and the repair of the self.* New York: W.W. Norton & Company.

[5] Begley, S. (2007). *Train your mind, change your brain: How a new science reveals our extraordinary potential to transform ourselves.* New York: Ballantine Books.

[6] Gurian, M. (2003). *The wonder of girls: Understanding the hidden natures of our daughters.* New York: Pocket Books.

[7] Brizendine, L. (2006). *The female brain.* New York: Morgan Road.

8 Brizendine, L. (2006). *The female brain.* New York: Morgan Road.

9 Brizendine, L. (2006). *The female brain.* New York: Morgan Road.

10 Brizendine, L. (2006). *The female brain.* New York: Morgan Road.

11 Taylor, S. (2003). *The tending instinct: Women, men, and the biology of relationships.* New York: Holt Paperbacks.

12 Taylor, S. (2003). *The tending instinct: Women, men, and the biology of relationships.* New York: Holt Paperbacks.

13 Taylor, S. (2003). *The tending instinct: Women, men, and the biology of relationships.* New York: Holt Paperbacks.

14 Gurian, M. (2003). *The wonder of girls: Understanding the hidden natures of our daughters.* New York: Pocket Books.

15 Nazario, B. (2005). *How male and female brains differ.* Retrieved on September 8, 2006, from http://www.medicinenet.com/script/main/art.asp?articlekey=50512

16 Brizendine, L. (2006). *The female brain.* New York: Morgan Road.

17 Gurian, M. (2003) *The wonder of girls: Understanding the hidden natures of our daughters.* New York: Pocket Books.

18 Tannen, D. (1990). *You just don't understand: Women and men in conversation.* New York: Ballantine. P. 76–77.

19 Tannen, D. (1990). *You just don't understand: Women and men in conversation.* New York: Ballantine. P. 77.

20 Gurian, M. (2003) *The wonder of girls: Understanding the hidden natures of our daughters.* New York: Pocket Books.

21 Brizendine, L. (2006). *The female brain.* New York: Morgan Road. P. 37.

22 Gilligan, C. (1982). *In a different voice: Psychological theory and women's development.* Cambridge, MA: Harvard University Press.

23 Baron-Cohen, S. (2003). *The essential difference: The truth about the male and female brain.* Basic Books, NY.

[24] Baron-Cohen, S. (2003). *The essential difference: The truth about the male and female brain.* Basic Books, NY.

[25] Brizendine, L. (2006). *The female brain.* New York: Morgan Road.

[26] Campbell, A. (1999). Staying alive: Evolution, culture, and women's intrasexual aggression. *Behavioral and Brain Sciences, 22,* 203–252.

[27] Campbell, A. (2002). *A mind of her own: The evolutionary psychology of women.* Oxford, UK: Oxford University Press.

[28] Brizendine, L. (2006). *The female brain.* New York: Morgan Road.

[29] Brizendine, L. (2006). *The female brain.* New York: Morgan Road.

[30] Panksepp, J. (2004). *Affective neuroscience: The foundations of human and animal emotions.* New York: Oxford University Press.

[31] Shapiro, F. & Maxfield, L. (2003). EMDR and information processing in psychotherapy treatment: Personal development and global implications. In D. J. Siegel & M. Solomon (Eds.), *Healing trauma: Attachment, mind, body, and brain.* New York: W.W. Norton and Company. P. 198.

[32] Shapiro, F. & Maxfield, L. (2003). EMDR and information processing in psychotherapy treatment: Personal development and global implications. In D. J. Siegel & M. Solomon (Eds.), *Healing trauma: Attachment, mind, body, and brain.* New York: W.W. Norton and Company. P. 201.

[33] Simmons, R. (2002). *Odd girl out: The hidden culture of girl's aggression.* NY: Harcourt Brace. P. 32.

[34] Gurian, M. (2003). *The wonder of girls: Understanding the hidden natures of our daughters.* New York: Pocket Books.

[35] Campbell, A. (1999). Staying alive: Evolution, culture, and women's intrasexual aggression. *Behavioral and Brain Sciences, 22,* 203–252.

[36] Campbell, A. (2002). *A mind of her own: The evolutionary psychology*

of women. Oxford, UK: Oxford University Press.

[37] Campbell, A. (1999). Staying alive: Evolution, culture, and women's intrasexual aggression. *Behavioral and Brain Sciences, 22*, 203–252.

[38] Campbell, A. (2002). *A mind of her own: The evolutionary psychology of women*. Oxford, UK: Oxford University Press.

[39] Campbell, A., Muncer, S., & Odher, J. (1997). Aggression and testosterone: Testing a biosocial model. *Aggressive behavior, 23*, 229–238.

[40] Etcoff, N. (1999). *Survival of the prettiest: The science of beauty.* New York: Doubleday.

CHAPTER IV: CATFIGHT! HOW THE MEDIA PORTRAYS AND TRIVIALIZES WOMEN

[1] American Psychological Association. (2007). *Report of the APA task force on the sexualization of girls.* Retrieved on January 5, 2008 from http://www.apa.org/pi/wpo/sexualizationrep.pdf

[2] *Television & health.* (n.d.). Retrieved June 1, 2008 from http://www.csun.edu/science/health/docs/tv&health.html

[3] Kilbourne, J. (2007, August). *Media and its effects on girls and women.* Interview conducted with Joan I. Rosenberg, Ph.D. and Erika Holiday, Psy.D., co-hosts of weekly radio show Women's Inspiration on KCSN.

[4] Hamilton, E. A., Mintz, L., & Kashubeck-West, S. (2007). Predictors of media effects on body dissatisfaction in European American women. *Sex Roles, 53*, 397–402.

[5] Lamb, S. & Mikel-Brown, L. (2006). *Packaging girlhood: Rescuing our daughters from marketer's schemes.* New York: St. Martin's Press.

[6] Durham, M. G. (2008). *The Lolita effect: The media sexualization of young girls and what we can do about it.* New York: Penguin Group.

[7] Kilbourne, J. (2007, August). *So sexy so soon: The sexualization*

of childhood. Invited address at the 115th annual convention of the American Psychological Association, San Francisco, CA.

8   American Psychological Association. (2007). *Report of the APA task force on the sexualization of girls.* Retrieved on January 5, 2008 from http://www.apa.org/pi/wpo/sexualizationrep.pdf

9   Gerbner, G., Gross, L., Morgan, M., & Signorielli, N. (1986). Living with television: The dynamics of the cultivation proves. In J. Bryant & D. Zillmann (Eds.), *Perspectives on media effects,* pp. 17– 40. Hillsdale, NJ: Lawrence Erlbaum Associates.

CHAPTER V: DAMNED IF YOU DO, DAMNED IF YOU DON'T

1   Heller, J.L. (1955). *Catch-22.* NY: Simon & Schuster.

2   Merriam-Webster. (2004). *The Merriam-Webster dictionary.* NY: Merriam-Webster.

3   Bateson, G. (1972). *Steps to an ecology of the mind.* New York: Ballantine.

4   Jamieson, K. H. (1995). *Beyond the double bind: Women and leadership.* New York: Oxford University Press, Inc.

5   Schaef. A.W. (1981). *Women's reality: An emerging female system in the white male society.* Minneapolis: Winston. P. 8.

6   Schaef. A.W. (1981). *Women's reality: An emerging female system in the white male society.* Minneapolis: Winston. P. 33.

7   Jamieson, K. H. (1995). *Beyond the double bind: Women and leadership.* New York: Oxford University Press, Inc.

8   Schaef. A.W. (1981). *Women's reality: An emerging female system in the white male society.* Minneapolis: Winston. P. 30.

9   Schaef. A.W. (1981). *Women's reality: An emerging female system in the white male society.* Minneapolis: Winston.

10 Birnbaum, D., Nosanchuk, T., & Croll. (1980). Children's stereotypes about sex differences in emotionality. *Sex Roles, 6,* 435–443.

[11] Saarni, C. (1988). Children's understanding of the interpersonal consequences of dissemblance of nonverbal emotional-expressive behavior. *Journal of Nonverbal Behavior, 12,* 275–294.

[12] Geer, C. G. & Shields, S. A. (1996). Women and emotion: Stereotypes and the double bind. In J. C. Chrisler, C. Golden, & P. D. Rozee (Eds.), *Lectures on the psychology of women,* pp. 356-373. NY: McGraw-Hill.

[13] Jamieson, K. H. (1995). *Beyond the double bind: Women and leadership.* New York: Oxford University Press, Inc. P. 80.

[14] Jamieson, K. H. (1995). *Beyond the double bind: Women and leadership.* New York: Oxford University Press, Inc.

[15] Jamieson, K. H. (1995). *Beyond the double bind: Women and leadership.* New York: Oxford University Press, Inc. p. 120–121.

[16] Jamieson, K. H. (1995). *Beyond the double bind: Women and leadership.* New York: Oxford University Press, Inc.

[17] Jamieson, K. H. (1995). *Beyond the double bind: Women and leadership.* New York: Oxford University Press, Inc.

[18] Goldberg, P. (1968). Are women prejudiced against women? *Transdash Action, 5,* 28–30.

[19] Paludi, M. A. & Bauer, W. D. (1983). Goldberg revisited: What's in an author's name? *Sex Roles: A Journal of Research, 9,* 3, 387–390.

[20] Paludi, M. A. & Strayer, L. A. (1985). What's in an author's name? Differential evaluations of performance as a function of authors name. *Sex Roles: A Journal of Research, 12,* 353–361.

[21] Cooley, C. H. ([1902] 1983). *Human Nature and the Social Order.* New York: Scribner's.

[22] Yeung, K. T. & Martin, J. L. (2003). The looking-glass self: An empirical test and elaboration. *Social Forces, 81,* 3, 843–879.

[23] Cox, D., Gosseling, C. & Robles, R. (2007, August). Double binds in women's experience of beauty and each other. In

J. I. Rosenberg (chair), *Diversity, culture and double binds: Dynamics compromising authenticity, well-being and relationships.* Symposium conducted at the 115th annual meeting of the American Psychological Association, San Francisco, CA.

[24] Cox, D.., Gosseling, C. & Robles, R. (2007, August). Double binds in women's experience of beauty and each other. In J. I. Rosenberg (chair), *Diversity, culture and double binds: Dynamics compromising authenticity, well-being and relationships.* Symposium conducted at the 115th annual meeting of the American Psychological Association, San Francisco, CA.

[25] Cox, D. (2007, May). *Dance of the beauty culture.* Interview conducted with Joan I. Rosenberg, Ph.D. and Erika Holiday, Psy.D., co-hosts of weekly radio show Women's Inspiration on KCSN.

[26] Broverman, I. K., Broverman, D. M., Clarkson, F. E., Rosenkrantz, P. S., & Vogel, S. R. (1970). Sex-role stereotypes and clinical judgments of mental health. *Journal of Consulting and Clinical Psychology, 34,* 1–7.

[27] Broverman, I. K., Broverman, D. M., Clarkson, F. E., Rosenkrantz, P. S., & Vogel, S. R. (1970). Sex-role stereotypes and clinical judgments of mental health. *Journal of Consulting and Clinical Psychology, 34,* 1–7.

[28] Seem, S. R. & Clark, M. D. (2006). Healthy women, healthy men, and healthy adults: An evaluation of gender role stereotypes in the twenty-first century. *Sex Roles: A Journal of Research.* P. 255.

[29] Seem, S. R. & Clark, M. D. (2006). Healthy women, healthy men, and healthy adults: An evaluation of gender role stereotypes in the twenty-first century. *Sex Roles: A Journal of Research.* P. 255.

[30] Seem, S. R. & Clark, M. D. (2006). Healthy women, healthy men, and healthy adults: An evaluation of gender role stereotypes in the twenty-first century. *Sex Roles: A Journal of Research.* P. 256.

31   Seem, S. R. & Clark, M. D. (2006). Healthy women, healthy men, and healthy adults: An evaluation of gender role stereotypes in the twenty-first century. *Sex Roles: A Journal of Research.* P. 257.

32   Jamieson, K. H. (1995). *Beyond the double bind: Women and leadership.* New York: Oxford University Press, Inc.

33   Zevy, L. (1999). Sexing the tomboy. In M. Rottnek (Ed.), *Sissies and tomboys: Gender nonconformity and homosexual childhood.* New York: NYU Press. Pp. 180–195.

34   Raimi, S., Raimi, I., Sargent, A. (Screenplay), & Raimi, S. (Director). (2007). *Spiderman III* [Motion picture]. United States: Columbia Pictures

35   Frost, M., France, M. (Screenplay), & Story, T. (Director). (2005). *Fantastic Four* [Motion picture]. United States: Twentieth Century Fox-Film Corporation

36   Sheerin, K. (Producer). (2005). *The Girls Next Door* [Television series]. United States: E! Entertainment

37   Schaef. A.W. (1981). *Women's reality: An emerging female system in the white male society.* Minneapolis: Winston.

38   Brown, L. M. (2003). *Girlfighting: Betrayal and rejection among girls.* New York, New York University Press. P. 201.

CHAPTER VI: BELONGING TO THE GIRLS CLUB: WHAT IT REALLY MEANS

1   Brown, L. M. (2003). *Girlfighting: Betrayal and rejection among girls.* New York, New York University Press. P. 37.

2   Kuhn, D., Nash, S. & Brucken, L. (1978). Sex-role of two and three-year-olds. *Child Development, 49,* 445–451.

3   Bem, S. L. (1993). *The lenses of gender: Transforming the debate on sexual inequality.* CT: Yale University Press.

4   Bem, S. L. (1993). *The lenses of gender: Transforming the debate on sexual inequality.* CT: Yale University Press. P. 2.

5   Bem, S. L. (1993). *The lenses of gender: Transforming the debate on sexual inequality.* CT: Yale University Press. P. 1.

[6] Schaef. A.W. (1981). *Women's reality: An emerging female system in the white male society.* Minneapolis: Winston.

[7] Bem, S. L. (1993). *The lenses of gender: Transforming the debate on sexual inequality.* CT: Yale University Press.

[8] Bem, S. L. (1993). *The lenses of gender: Transforming the debate on sexual inequality.* CT: Yale University Press.

[9] Bem, S. L. (1993). *The lenses of gender: Transforming the debate on sexual inequality.* CT: Yale University Press.

[10] Bem, S. L. (1993). *The lenses of gender: Transforming the debate on sexual inequality.* CT: Yale University Press.

[11] Daniels, C. (2007). *Ghettonation: A journey into the land of bling and home of the shameless.* New York: Doubleday.

[12] Bem, S. L. (1993). *The lenses of gender: Transforming the debate on sexual inequality.* CT: Yale University Press. P. 149.

[13] Bem, S. L. (1993). *The lenses of gender: Transforming the debate on sexual inequality.* CT: Yale University Press. P. 192–194.

[14] Bem, S. L. (1993). *The lenses of gender: Transforming the debate on sexual inequality.* CT: Yale University Press.

[15] F. Rabinowitz, M. Engler-Carlson & M. Kiselica (personal communication, June 2, 2007)

[16] Bem, S. L. (1981). Gender schema theory: A cognitive account of sex-typing. *Psychological Review, 88,* 354–364.

CHAPTER VII: OPPRESSIVE EXPERIENCES

[1] Heilman, M. (2001). Description and prescription: How gender stereotypes prevent women's ascent up the organizational ladder. *Journal of Social Issues, 57,* 657–674.

[2] Prentice, D. A. & Carranza, E. (2002). What women and men should be, shouldn't be, are allowed to be, and don't' have to be: The contents of prescriptive gender stenotypes. *Psychology of Women Quarterly, 26,* 269–281.

[3] Eagly, A. & Karau, S. J. (2002). Role congruity theory of prejudice toward female leaders. *Psychological Review, 109,* 573–598.

[4] Gardner, W. L., Pickett, C. L., & Brewer, M. B. (2000). Social exclusion and selective memory: How the need to belong influences memory for social events. *Personality and Social Psychology Bulletin, 26*, 486–496.

[5] Heim, P., Murphy, S. & Golant, S. (2001). *In the company of women. Indirect aggression among women: Why we hurt each other and how to stop.* New York: Penguin Group, Inc.

[6] Goodwin, M. H. (2002). Exclusion in girls' peer groups: Ethnographic analysis of language practices on the playground. *Human Development, 45*, 392–415.

[7] Caplan, P. J. (2000). *Don't blame mother: Mending the mother-daughter relationship.* United Kingdom: Routledge. P. 97–98.

[8] Chesler, P. (2003). *Women's inhumanity to woman.* New York: Nation Books.

CHAPTER VIII: COMPETITION AND AGGRESSION

[1] Buss, A. H. (1961). *The psychology of aggression.* New York: John Wiley & Sons, Inc.

[2] Keenan, E. & Shaw, D. (1997). Developmental and social influences on young girls' early problem behaviors. *Psychological Bulletin, 121*, 95–113.

[3] Gilligan, C. (1982). *In a different voice: Psychological theory and women's development.* Cambridge, MA: Harvard University Press.

[4] Simmons, R. (2002). *Odd girl out: The hidden culture of girl's aggression.* NY: Harcourt Brace.

[5] Tannenbaum, L. (2002). *Catfight: Rivalries among women – from diets to dating, from the boardroom to the delivery room.* New York: Seven Stories Press.

[6] Rock, C. (Screenplay), & Gallen, J. (Director). (2004). *Never scared* [Comedy Special]. United States: Home Box Office (HBO)

[7] Shapiro-Barash, S. (2006). *Tripping the prom queen: The truth*

about women and rivalry. New York: St. Martin's Press.

8   Cox, D., Gosseling, C., & Robles, R. (2007). Double binds in women's experience of beauty and each other. In J. I. Rosenberg (chair), D*iversity, culture and double binds: Dynamics compromising authenticity, well-being and relationships.* Symposium conducted at the 115th annual meeting of the American Psychological Association, San Francisco, CA.

9   Cox, D., Gosseling, C., & Robles, R. (2007). Double binds in women's experience of beauty and each other. In J. I. Rosenberg (chair), D*iversity, culture and double binds: Dynamics compromising authenticity, well-being and relationships.* Symposium conducted at the 115th annual meeting of the American Psychological Association, San Francisco, CA.

10   Tannenbaum, L. (2002). *Catfight: Rivalries among women – from diets to dating, from the boardroom to the delivery room.* New York: Seven Stories Press.

CHAPTER IX: BUILDING COLLABORATIVE RELATIONSHIPS AND COMMUNITY

1   Michael, Y. L., Colditz, G. A., Coakley, E., & Kawachi, I. (1999). Health behaviors, social networks, and healthy aging: Cross-sectional evidence from the nurses' health study. *Quality of Life Research, 8,* 711–722.

2   Brown, L. M. (2003). *Girlfighting: Betrayal and rejection among girls.* New York, NYU Press. P. 47.

3   Brown, L. M. (2003). *Girlfighting: Betrayal and rejection among girls.* New York, NYU Press. P. 216–217.

4   Brown, L. M. (2003). *Girlfighting: Betrayal and rejection among girls.* New York, NYU Press. P. 217.

5   Brown, L. M. (2003). *Girlfighting: Betrayal and rejection among girls.* New York, NYU Press. P. 212–213.

6   Jamieson, K. H. (1995). *Beyond the double bind: Women and leadership.* New York: Oxford University Press, Inc. P. 190–197.

[7] Brown, L. M. (2003). *Girlfighting: Betrayal and rejection among girls.* New York, NYU Press. P. 222.

[8] Kilbourne, J. (2007, August). *Media and its effect on girls and women.* Interview conducted with Joan I. Rosenberg, Ph.D. and Erika Holiday, Psy.D. co-hosts of weekly radio show Women's Inspiration on KCSN.

[9] Media literacy skills. Retrieved June 2, 2008, from www. nmmlp. org

[10] Media literacy skills. Retrieved June 2, 2008, from www. nmmlp. org

[11] Media literacy skills. Retrieved January 3, 2009, from http://nmmlp.org/media_literacy/deconstructing_media. html

[12] Anderson, C. (2007, April). *Effects of media violence.* Interview conducted with Joan I. Rosenberg, Ph.D. and Erika Holiday, Psy.D., co-hosts of weekly radio show Women's Inspiration on KCSN.

[13] Anderson, C. A., Gentile, D. A., & Buckley, K. E. (2007). *Violent video game effects on children and adolescence: Theory, research and public policy.* London: Oxford University Press.

[14] Franklin, A. J. (1999). Invisibility syndrome and racial identity development in psychotherapy and counseling African American men. *The Counseling Psychologist,* 27, 6, 761–793. p. 764. (Antithesis of Invisibility Syndrome as described by A. J. Franklin).

References

American Psychological Association. (2007). *Report of the APA task force on the sexualization of girls.* Retrieved on January 5, 2008 from http://www.apa.org/pi/wpo/sexualizationrep.pdf

Anderson, C. (2007, April). *Effects of media violence.* Interview conducted with Joan I. Rosenberg, Ph.D. and Erika Holiday, Psy.D., co-hosts of weekly radio show Women's Inspiration on KCSN.

Anderson, C. A., Gentile, D. A., & Buckley, K. E. (2007). *Violent video game effects on children and adolescence: Theory, research and public policy.* London: Oxford University Press.

Archer, J., & Coyne, S. M. (2005). An integrated review of indirect, relational, and social aggression. *Personality and Social Psychology Review, 9,* (3), 212–230.

Baron-Cohen, S. (2003). *The essential difference: The truth about the male and female brain.* New York: Basic Books.

Bateson, G. (1972). *Steps to an ecology of the mind.* New York: Ballantine.

Begley, S. (2007). *Train your mind, change your brain: How a new science reveals our extraordinary potential to transform ourselves.* New York: Ballantine Books.

Bem, S. L. (1981). Gender schema theory: A cognitive account of sex-typing. *Psychological Review, 88,* 354–364.

Bem, S. L. (1983). Gender schema theory and its implications for child development: Raising gender-aschematic children in a gender-schematic society. *Signs: Journal of Women in Culture and Society, 8,* 598–616.

Bem, S. L. (1993). *The lenses of gender: Transforming the debate on sexual inequality.* CT: Yale University Press.

Bem, S. L. (1995). Dismantling gender polarization and compulsory heterosexuality: Should we turn the volume down or up? *The Journal of Sex Research, 32*(4), 329–334.

Birnbaum, D., Nosanchuk, T., & Croll. (1980). Children's

stereotypes about sex differences in emotionality. *Sex Roles,* *6,* 435–443.

Björkqvist, K. (1994). Sex differences in physical, verbal, and indirect aggression: A review of recent research. *Sex Roles, 30,* 177–188.

Björkqvist, K., Österman, K., & Kaukiainen A. (1992). The development of direct and indirect aggressive strategies in males and females. In K. Björkqvist & P. Niemelä (Eds.), *Of mice and women: Aspects of female aggression* (pp. 51–64). San Diego, CA: Academic Press.

Björkqvist, K. Österman, K., Lagerspetz, K. M. J., Landau, S. F., Caprara, G. V., & Fraczek, A. (2001). Aggression, victimization, and sociometric status: Findings from Finland, Israel, Italy, and Poland. In Ramirez, M. & Richardson, D. S. (Eds.), *Cross-cultural approaches to research on aggression and reconciliation* (pp. 111–119). Huntington, NY: Nova Science Publishers.

Brizendine, L. (2006). *The female brain.* New York: Morgan Road.

Broverman, I. K., Broverman, D. M., Clarkson, F. E., Rosenkrantz, P. S., & Vogel, S. R. (1970). Sex-role stereotypes and clinical judgments of mental health. *Journal of Consulting and Clinical Psychology,* 34, 1–7.

Brown, L. M. (2003). *Girlfighting: Betrayal and rejection among girls.* New York: New York University Press.

Buss, A. H. (1961). *The psychology of aggression.* New York: John Wiley & Sons, Inc.

Cairns, R. B., Cairns, B. D., Neckerman, H. J., Ferguson, L. L., & Gariepy, J. L. (1989). Growth & aggression I: Childhood to early adolescence. *Developmental Psychology, 25,* 320–330.

Campbell, A. (1999). Staying alive: Evolution, culture, and women's intrasexual aggression. *Behavioral and Brain Sciences, 22,* 203–252.

Campbell, A. (2002). *A mind of her own: The evolutionary psychology of women.* Oxford, UK: Oxford University Press.

Campbell, A., Muncer, S., & Odher, J. (1997). Aggression and testosterone: Testing a biosocial model. *Aggressive behavior, 23*, 229–238.

Campbell, A.S., Shirley, L. & Caygill, L. (2002). Sex-typed preferences in three domains: Do two-year-olds need cognitive variables? *British Journal of Psychology, 93*, 2, 203–217.

Caplan, P. J. (2000). *Don't blame mother: Mending the mother-daughter relationship.* United Kingdom: Routledge. pp. 97–98.

Casey-Cannon, S., Hayward, C., & Gowen, K. (2001). Middle-school girl's reports of peer victimization: Concerns, consequences, and implications. *Professional School Counseling, 5*, 138–144

Celizic, M. (2008). *Teens videotape beating as revenge for online posts.* Retrieved June 2, 2008, from http://www.msnbc.msn.com/id/24009077/

Chesler, P. (2002). *Woman's inhumanity to woman.* NY: Nation Books.

Chu, J. (2005). You wanna take this online? Cyberspace is the 21st century bully's playgroup where girls play rougher than boys. *Time*, Vol. 166, 6.

Conway, A. (2005). Girls, aggression, and emotion regulation. *American Journal of Orthopsychiatry, 75*, 2.

Cooley, C. H. ([1902] 1983). *Human Nature and the Social Order.* New York: Scribner's.

Cox, D., Gosseling, C., & Robles, R. (2007). Double binds in women's experience of beauty and each other. In J. I. Rosenberg (chair), D*iversity, culture and double binds: Dynamics compromising authenticity, well-being and relationships.* Symposium conducted at the 115th annual meeting of the American Psychological Association, San Francisco, CA.

Cox, D. (2007, May). *Dance of the beauty culture.* Interview conducted with Joan I. Rosenberg, Ph.D and Erika Holiday, Psy.D., co-hosts of weekly radio show Women's Inspiration on KCSN.

Crick, N. R. (1996). The role of overt aggression, relational aggression, and prosocial behavior in children's social adjustment. *Child Development, 33*, 610–617.

Crick, N. R., & Grotpeter, J. K. (1995). Relational aggression, gender, and social-psychological adjustment. *Child Development, 66*, 710–722.

Crick, N. R., & Grotpeter, J. K. (1996). Children's treatment by peers: Victims of relational and overt aggression. *Development and Psychopathology, 8*, 367–380.

Crick, N. R., Werner, N. E., Casas, J. F., O'Brien, K. M., Nelson, D. A., Grotpeter, J. K., & Markon, K. (1999). Childhood aggression and gender: A new look at an old problem. In D. Bernstein et al. (Eds.), *Gender and motivation: Nebraska symposium on motivation* (Vol. 45; pp. 75–141). Lincoln, NE: University of Nebraska Press.

Daniels, C. (2007). *Ghettonation: A journey into the land of bling and home of the shameless.* New York: Doubleday.

Durham, M. G. (2008). *The Lolita effect: The media sexualization of young girls and what we can do about it.* New York: Penguin Group.

Eagly, A. & Karau, S.J. (2002). Role congruity theory of prejudice toward female leaders. *Psychological Review, 109*, 573–598

Etcoff, N. (1999). *Survival of the prettiest: The science of beauty.* New York: Doubleday.

Fey, T. (Screenplay), & Waters, M. (Director). (2004). *Mean girls* [Motion picture]. United States: Paramount Pictures.

Franklin, A.J. (1999). Invisibility syndrome and racial identity development in psychotherapy and counseling African American men. *The Counseling Psychologist*, 27, 6, 761–793.

Frost, M., France, M. (Screenplay), & Story, T. (Director). (2005). *Fantastic Four* [Motion picture]. United States: Twentieth Century Fox-Film Corporation.

Galen, B.R., & Underwood, M.K. (1997). A developmental investigation of social aggression among children. *Developmental Psychology, 33*, 589–600.

Gardner, W. L., Pickett, C. L. & Brewer, M. B. (2000). Social exclusion and selective memory: How the need to belong influences memory for social events. *Personality and Social Psychology Bulletin, 26,* 486–496.

Geer, C. G. & Shields, S. A. (1996). Women and emotion: Stereotypes and the double bind. In J. C. Chrisler, C. Golden, & P. D. Rozee (Eds.), *Lectures on the psychology of women.* NY: McGraw-Hill. 356–373.

Gerbner, G., Gross, L., Morgan, M., & Signorielli, N. (1986). Living with television: The dynamics of the cultivation proves. In J. Bryant & D. Zillmann (Eds.), *Perspectives on media effects,* pp. 17–40. Hillsdale, NJ: Lawrence Erlbaum Associates.

Gilligan, C. (1982). *In a different voice: Psychological theory and women's development.* Cambridge, MA: Harvard University Press.

Goldberg, P. (1968). Are women prejudiced against women? *Transdash Action, 5,* 28–30.

Goodwin, M. H. (2002). Exclusion in girls' peer groups: Ethnographic analysis of language practices on the playground. *Human Development, 45,* 392–415.

Gray, K. (2006). *How mean can teens be? "Primetime" special shows how the internet can fuel bullying and fighting.* Retrieved October 12, 2006, from http://abcnews.go.com/Primetime/story?id=2421562&page=1

Gurian, M. (2003). *The wonder of girls: Understanding the hidden natures of our daughters.* New York: Pocket Books.

Gurian, M. (2007, February). *The wonder of girls.* Interview conducted with Joan I. Rosenberg, Ph.D. and Erika Yomtobian, Psy.D., co-hosts of weekly radio show Women's Inspiration on KCSN.

Hamilton, E.A., Mintz, L., & Kashubeck-West, S. (2007). Predictors of media effects on body dissatisfaction in European American women. *Sex Roles,* Vol. 53, 397–402.

Harrell, S. (2000). A multidimensional conceptualization of racism-related stress: Implications for the well-being of people of color. *Journal of Orthopsychiatry, 70*(1), 42–57.

Heilman, M. (2001). Description and prescription: How gender stereotypes prevent women's ascent up the organizational ladder. *Journal of Social Issues, 57,* 657–674.

Heim, P., Murphy, S., & Golant, S. (2001). *In the company of women. Indirect aggression among women: Why we hurt each other and how to stop.* New York: Penguin Group, Inc.

Heller, J.L. (1955). *Catch-22.* New York: Simon & Schuster.

Jamieson, K.H. (1995). *Beyond the double bind: Women and leadership.* New York: Oxford University Press, Inc.

Jost, J. (1997). An experimental replication of the depressed-entitlement effect among women. *Psychology of Women Quarterly, 21,* 387–393.

Keenan, E. & Shaw, D. (1997). Developmental and social influences on young girls' early problem behaviors. *Psychological Bulletin, 121,* 95–113.

Kilbourne, J. (2007, August). *So sexy so soon: The sexualization of childhood.* Invited address at the 115th annual convention of the American Psychological Association, San Francisco, CA.

Kilbourne, J. (2007, August). *Media and its effect on girls and women.* Interview conducted with Joan I. Rosenberg, Ph.D. and Erika Holiday, Psy.D., co-hosts of weekly radio show Women's Inspiration on KCSN.

Kuhn, D., Nash, S. & Brucken, L. (1978). Sex-role of two and three-year olds. *Child Development, 49,* 445–451.

Ladd, B. K., & Ladd, G. W. (2001). *Variations in peer victimization: Relations in peer maladjustment.* In J. Juvonen & S. Graham (Eds.), Peer harassment in school: The plight of the vulnerable and victimized (p. 25–48). New York: Guildford Press.

Lagerspetz, K. M. J., Bjorkqvist, K., & Peltonen, T. (1988). Is indirect aggression typical of females? Gender differences in aggressiveness in 11- to 12-year-old children. *Aggressive*

Behavior, 14, 403–414.

Lamb, S. (2002). *The secret lives of girls: What good girls really do – sex play, aggression, and their guilt.* New York: The Free Press (Simon and Schuster).

Lamb, S. & Mikel-Brown, L. (2006). *Packaging girlhood: Rescuing our daughters from marketer's schemes.* New York: St. Martin's Press.

Levin, D. E., & Kilbourne, J. (2008). *So sexy, so soon: The new sexualized childhood and what parents can do to protect their kids.* New York: Ballantine Books.

Lutz, K. M., & Smith, K. (Screenplay) & Wolf, F. (Director). (2008). *The house bunny* [Motion Picture]. United States: Happy Madison Productions.

Media literacy Skills. Retrieved June 2, 2008, from www.nmmlp. org

Merriam-Webster. (2004). *The Merriam-Webster dictionary.* New York: Merriam-Webster.

Michael, Y. L., Colditz, G. A., Coakley, E., & Kawachi, I. (1999). Health behaviors, social networks, and healthy aging: Cross-sectional evidence from the nurses' health study. *Quality of Life Research, 8,* 711–722.

Mills, R.S.L., & Rubin, K.H. (1992). A longitudinal study of maternal beliefs about children's social behavior. *Merrill-Palmer Quarterly, 38,* 494–512.

National Crime Prevention Council. (2003). Bullying, not terrorist attack, biggest threat seen by U.S. teens. Washington, DC: (press release).

Nazario, B. (2005). *How male and female brains differ.* Retrieved on September 8, 2006, from http://www.medicinenet.com/script/main/art.asp?articlekey=50512

Pajares, F. & Schunk, D.H. (2002). Self and self-belief in psychology and education: A historical perspective (p. 6). In J. Aronson & D. Cordova (Eds.), *Improving academic achievement: Impact of psychological factors on education,* (p. 3–21), New York:

Academic Press.

Paludi, M. A. & Bauer, W. D. (1983). Goldberg revisited: What's in an author's name? *Sex Roles: A Journal of Research*, *9*, 3, 387–390.

Paludi, M. A. & Strayer, L. A. (1985). What's in an author's name? Different evaluations of performance as a function of author's name. *Sex Roles: A Journal of Research*, *12*, 353–361.

Panksepp, J. (2004). *Affective neuroscience: The foundations of human and animal emotions*. New York: Oxford University Press.

Perry, D.G., Perry, L.C., & Weiss, R.J. (1989). Sex differences in the consequences that children anticipate for aggression. *Developmental Psychology*, *25*, 312–319.

Prentice, D.A. & Carranza, E. (2002). What women and men should be, shouldn't be, are allowed to be, and don't' have to be: The contents of prescriptive gender stenotypes. *Psychology of Women Quarterly*, *26*, 269–281.

Prothrow-Stith, D., & Spivak, H.R. (2005) *Sugar and spice and no longer nice: How we can stop girls' violence*. New York: Jossey-Bass.

Raimi, S., Raimi, I., Sargent, A. (Screenplay), & Raimi, S. (Director). (2007). *Spiderman 3* [Motion picture]. United States: Columbia Pictures

Rock, C. (Screenplay), & Gallen, J. (Director). (2004). *Never scared* [Comedy Special]. United States: Home Box Office (HBO).

Saarni, C. (1988). Children's understanding of the interpersonal consequences of dissemblance of nonverbal emotional-expressive behavior. *Journal of Nonverbal Behavior*, *12*, 275–294.

Schaef. A.W. (1981). *Women's reality: An emerging female system in the white male society*. Minneapolis: Winston.

Schore, A. (2003). *Affect regulation and the repair of the self*. New York: W.W. Norton & Company.

Seem, S. R. & Clark, M. D. (2006). Healthy women, healthy men, and healthy adults: An evaluation of gender role stereotypes in the twenty-first century. *Sex-roles: A Journal of Research, 55,* 247–258.

Shapiro, F. & Maxfield, L. (2003). EMDR and information processing in psychotherapy treatment: Personal development and global implications. In D. J. Siegel & M. Solomon (Eds.), *Healing trauma: Attachment, mind, body, and brain.* New York: W.W. Norton and Company.

Shapiro-Barash, S. (2006). *Tripping the prom queen: The truth about women and rivalry.* New York: St. Martin's Press.

Sheerin, K. (Producer). (2005). *The Girls Next Door* [Television series]. United States: E! Entertainment.

Siegel, D. J. (1999). *The developing mind: Toward a neurobiology of interpersonal experience.* New York: The Guilford Press.

Siegel, D. J. (2007). *The mindful brain: Reflection and attunement in the cultivation of well-being.* New York: W.W. Norton & Company.

Simmons, R. (2002). *Odd girl out: The hidden culture of girl's aggression.* New York: Harcourt Brace.

Sue, D. W. & Sue, D. (2003). *Counseling the culturally diverse: Theory and practice.* New York: John Wiley & Sons, Inc.

Sue, D. W., Capodilup, C. M., Torino, G. C., Bucceri, J. M., Holder, A. M. B., Nadal, K. L., & Esquilin, M. (2007). Racial microaggressions in everyday life: Implications for clinical practice. *American Psychologist, 62,* 271–286.

Tannen, D. (1990). *You just don't understand: Women and men in conversation.* New York: Ballantine.

Tannenbaum, L. (2002). *Catfight: Rivalries among women - from diets to dating, from the boardroom to the delivery room.* New York: Seven Stories Press.

Taylor, S. (2003). *The tending instinct: Women, men, and the biology of relationships.* New York: Holt Paperbacks.

Television & health. (n.d.). Retrieved June 1, 2008 from http://www.csun.edu/science/health/docs/tv&health.html

Underwood, M. K. (2003). *Social aggression among girls.* New York: Guilford Press.

Wiredsafety.org- *The world's largest internet safety and help group* (n.d.). Retrieved July 13, 2008 from http://www.wiredsafety.org/

Wiseman, R. (2002). *Queen bees and wannabees: Helping your daughter survive cliques, gossip, boyfriends and other realities of adolescence.* New York: Crown Publishers.

Yeung, K. T. & Martin, J. L. (2003). The looking-glass self: An empirical test and elaboration. *Social Forces, 81*, 3, 843–879.

Yomtobian, E. (2005). *A theoretical model of women oppressing women: Contextual factors, psychological processes and the developmental trajectory.* Unpublished doctoral thesis, Phillips Graduate Institute, Encino, CA.

Zevy, L. (1999). Sexing the tomboy. In M. Rottnek (Eds.), *Sissies and tomboys: Gender nonconformity and homosexual childhood.* New York: NYU Press.

5 key questions. (2002–2007). Retrieved June 2, 2008, from http://www.medialit.org

The Next Step . . .

1. To book Dr. Erika Holiday and/or Dr. Joan I. Rosenberg for your organization's or agency's next event and experience their dynamic keynotes and seminars
    *   for Dr. Holiday, visit: www.drerikaholiday.com or call 818-512-4093, and
    *   for Dr. Rosenberg, visit: www.drjrosenberg.com or call 310-477-3242
2. Invest in your group's or organization's continuing diversity education or workplace training and receive discounts on bulk purchases of *Mean Girls, Meaner Women*
    *   Email us at www.meangirlsmeanerwomen.com for more information
3. Go to www.meangirlsmeanerwomen.com to:
    *   Receive your complimentary report, "Tips for Creating Closer Connections between Women"
    *   Sign up for our free e-newsletter
    *   See links to other helpful resources
    *   Sign up for our free e-zine
4. Mean Girls, Meaner Women is also available in audio format
5. *Questions? Comments? Stories to tell? Or to arrange consulting, speaking or training events or other programs, email or call us at the numbers above.*

About the Authors

ERIKA HOLIDAY, Psy.D., is a California-licensed psychologist. She has a private psychotherapy practice in Los Angeles, California, and her specialty areas include relationship issues; grief and loss; matters related to health; women's issues; and issues related to all aspects of diversity. She is a highly sought professional speaker especially for presentations and workshops on diversity and how teens, women and men can create healthier relationships. Dr. Holiday serves as co-host of *Full Circle*, a weekly radio program in Los Angeles on KCSN/88.5 FM / (kcsn.org), a program dedicated to promoting a more positive culture. Additionally she serves as part-time faculty at Pierce and Valley Community Colleges in Los Angeles.

JOAN I. ROSENBERG, Ph.D., a California-licensed psychologist, is an acclaimed national public speaker, trainer and consultant who co-hosts *Full Circle*, a weekly radio program in Los Angeles on KCSN/88.5 FM (kcsn.org), a program dedicated to promoting a more positive culture. Dr. Rosenberg speaks and conducts trainings and programs on such topics as suicide prevention, eating disorders, addiction prevention, diversity and multiculturalism, building positive relationships using recent discoveries about the brain, and a variety of men's and women's issues. She maintains an independent psychotherapy practice in Los Angeles, CA. She served as a Staff Psychologist at the University of California, Los Angeles, and has taught in masters and doctoral programs at the University of Southern California, Pepperdine University, Wright State University, and Phillips Graduate Institute.

Made in the USA
Lexington, KY
10 October 2012